Building Professional
Nursing Communication

Establishing and building effective relationships are essential skills for safe nursing practice. *Building Professional Nursing Communication* guides students through the concepts integral to successful communication for nurses.

Each chapter addresses communication theory and clearly demonstrates how it can be applied both to university studies and to professional nursing practice. Learning is extended further through case studies, practical scenarios and student learning activities. The book also addresses recent developments in online learning, covering information literacy, digital learning and consultation, as well as emerging forms of digital communication such as e-portfolios, blogs and new media.

This book brings together authors from nursing and communication backgrounds, combining extensive research and practical experience in both fields. This diverse team mirrors the interdisciplinary nature of the nursing role in the contemporary healthcare sector.

A companion website contains links to video and audio resources, and provides learning activities to connect these to the book's content. These resources can be accessed at www.cambridge.edu.au/academic/nursingcommunication.

Building Professional Nursing Communication is an essential resource for nursing students throughout their entire degree.

Jill Lawrence is Professor of Communication and Associate Dean (Students) in the Faculty of Business, Education, Law and Arts at the University of Southern Queensland.

Cheryl Perrin is Associate Professor in the School of Nursing and Midwifery at the University of Southern Queensland.

Eleanor Kiernan is Lecturer, Communication, in the Faculty of Business, Education, Law and Arts at the University of Southern Queensland.

Building
Professional
Nursing
Communication

Edited by

Jill Lawrence *Cheryl Perrin* *Eleanor Kiernan*

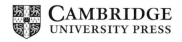

CAMBRIDGE
UNIVERSITY PRESS

CAMBRIDGE
UNIVERSITY PRESS

University Printing House, Cambridge CB2 8BS, United Kingdom

One Liberty Plaza, 20th Floor, New York, NY 10006, USA

477 Williamstown Road, Port Melbourne, VIC 3207, Australia

314–321, 3rd Floor, Plot 3, Splendor Forum, Jasola District Centre, New Delhi – 110025, India

79 Anson Road, #06–04/06, Singapore 079906

Cambridge University Press is part of the University of Cambridge.

It furthers the University's mission by disseminating knowledge in the pursuit of education, learning and research at the highest international levels of excellence.

www.cambridge.org
Information on this title: www.cambridge.org/9781107470460

© Cambridge University Press 2015

First published 2015 (version 3, December 2018)

Cover designed by Eggplant Communications
Typeset by Aptara Corp.
Printed in Singapore by Markono Print Media Pte Ltd, October 2018

A catalogue record for this publication is available from the British Library

A Cataloguing-in-Publication entry is available from the catalogue of the National Library of Australia at www.nla.gov.au

ISBN 978-1-107-47046-0 Paperback

Additional resources for this publication at
www.cambridge.edu.au/academic/nursingcommunication

Every effort has been made in preparing this book to provide accurate and up-to-date information that is in accord with accepted standards and practice at the time of publication. Although case histories are drawn from actual cases, every effort has been made to disguise the identities of the individuals involved. Nevertheless, the authors, editors and publishers can make no warranties that the information contained herein is totally free from error, not least because clinical standards are constantly changing through research and regulation. The authors, editors and publishers therefore disclaim all liability for direct or consequential damages resulting from the use of material contained in this book. Readers are strongly advised to pay careful attention to information provided by the manufacturer of any drugs or equipment that they plan to use.

Permission: Kossen, Kiernan & Lawrence 2011 text and artwork in Chapters 3, 4 and 5 reproduced with permission from Chris Kossen, Eleanor Kiernan and Jill Lawrence, *Communicating for Success* © 2014 Pearson Australia. Figure 8.1 © shutterstock.com / snapgalleria.

Foreword

The first female Prime Minister of Australia, Julia Gillard, recognised the value of nurses, whom she described as the 'backbone' of the health system. I agree with her profoundly. My experiences as a nurse, as a nurse teacher and researcher, and indeed as a patient and as a family member of a patient, have all demonstrated the centrality of nurses as the accessible communicator.

Nurses 'make sense' of the health system and indeed of healthcare; patients and families look to nurses to tell them what's happening, in everyday language they can understand. Nurses are also at the centre of the healthcare team, and spend much of their time ensuring that other health professionals are up to date with what's happening for their patients.

At the heart of nursing, then, is the capacity to make connections: to communicate clearly, deeply and meaningfully. It is also the capacity to communicate accurately, succinctly and effectively with other members of the health team. It's the ability to write and keep accurate records. And finally it's the capacity to advocate for and on behalf of patients and their families, and to ensure adequate resourcing is made available.

Communication might seem a natural skill, but there is plenty of evidence to suggest that it's not inborn for many health workers. Communication can and must be taught; yet it's challenging to do so. Not least because everyone assumes they can communicate and may not realise their challenges in this space!

That's where this visionary Australian text, designed specifically for nurses, will make a significant impact. This text recognises the extent and variety of communication skills required each and every day by nurses; and responds by providing nurses with the essential knowledge they will need to be effective communicators. A variety of nursing authors, together with communications experts, have written accessible and contemporary chapters that explore the key areas of communication practice for nurses.

I commend the editors and authors of this work for their vision, expertise and passion to share their knowledge with nurses and nursing students. I commend this book to all nursing students, nurses and indeed all health professionals.

Cath Rogers
Head of School of Nursing
University of Southern Queensland

Foreword

Paradigms of nursing are many and varied, and differ greatly across the world. This fact is never more important then when considering communication in the context of professional care. This important text acknowledges the skill of communication as pivotal to the role of the nurse. Paradigms of nursing have shifted over time, and with increased autonomy and, more recently, assumed leadership of the multi-disciplinary team, communication has never been more important.

For many decades student nurses were taught only what they needed to know in order to carry out their role; higher level problem-solving skills being associated with others educated to a different blueprint. This, of course, relates to the previously mentioned paradigms of nursing or particular world-views. Over recent decades two different views have been recognised. The first of these sees nursing as a collection of procedures, requiring some skill but being initiated and directed predominantly by doctors, while the second views nursing as a particular kind of interpersonal interaction that has specific goals determined by the nurse, and uses clinical judgement based upon specific nursing knowledge. Communication is pivotal to the second conceptualisation and is therefore an important facet of nurse education.

If nurses are to belong to, and lead, multi-disciplinary teams they must be comfortable acting as the integrating force between professionals and families. Communication skills must be developed to a high level to allow this to happen and this book facilitates that development. Communication theory is explicitly addressed and repeatedly applied to the clinical situation allowing students to explicate their experiences and continually develop their practice.

This book will complement pre-registration studies in Australia and beyond, and be a useful reflective companion for the registered nurse for many years to come. I commend the editors and authors for their authentic approach and encourage nurses everywhere to embrace and apply the content of this very important text.

Lyn Karstadt
Executive Dean (Health, Engineering and Sciences)
University of Southern Queensland

Contents

7   Digital skills in healthcare practice   **155**

Clint Moloney and Helen Farley

8   Professional skills for nurses and other health professionals: Contexts and capability of practice   **182**

Cheryl Perrin, David Stanley and Melissa Taylor

**9   Contributing to evidence-based healthcare cultures
        through lifelong learning   205**

Lisa Beccaria, Clint Moloney and Craig Lockwood

1 Communication in context: Developing a professional identity

Nicholas Ralph

Learning objectives

- Establish and identify foundations for effective professional communication.
- Develop insights into the role of self-awareness and its relationship to developing a professional identity.
- Recognise and reflect on the professional requirements inherent to nursing.
- Identify pathways to professional practice and professional development.
- Critically explore the change and challenges present in the evolving healthcare contexts.

Key terms

- Accreditation
- Competence
- Emotional intelligence
- Professional identity

Introduction

Communication refers to the act of imparting or exchanging information by speaking, writing or using some other medium (Arnold & Boggs, 2013). Because it is a routine part of life, it is easy for the importance of effective communication to be forgotten. However, its benefits have been demonstrated in every aspect of modern life, such as enhanced safety in aviation (Leonard, Graham & Bonacum, 2004), improved business management practices (Kernbach, Eppler & Bresciani, 2014) and instant, accurate information on developing world events (Veil, Buehner & Palenchar, 2011).

In nursing and healthcare, effective communication is necessary for delivering safe nursing care, as it reduces the risk of harm to the patient, enhances clinical outcomes and encourages reflective practice among clinicians (Haynes et al., 2011; Lin et al., 2013). Poor communication is known to affect the quality and safety of nursing care delivery (Hughes & Mitchell, 2008; Mills, Neily & Dunn, 2008). Throughout this book, you will be guided through concepts that are integral to effective communication. However, in this chapter we explore the person at the centre of all the communication you will experience as a registered nurse: you. In developing an awareness of the contexts of communication, it is important to address the role of self, professional identity and professional awareness. Having a strong sense of your professional identity provides a useful foundation for effectively communicating throughout your nursing career. Furthermore, scoping the unique characteristics you bring to nursing will help you understand the similarly unique perspectives of others with whom you may study or work, or those for whom you care. You will soon realise that developing your professional identity and becoming self-aware are necessary to function ethically and professionally in the nursing role. Before long, you will likely face situations that may encroach on your personal values, and demand an ethical and professional response – however difficult that may be.

Navigating the complexities of the healthcare environment is always challenging, whether it involves communicating with patients to assess the extent of their condition or communicating with a grieving family whose loved one is dying. Developing your professional identity through improved self-awareness will enhance your ability to:

- communicate ethically and professionally
- articulate your motivations in nursing
- employ strategies for reflective practice, and
- heighten your understanding of the nursing profession.

Understanding the nursing profession will also be useful for establishing insight into how it communicates its defining features, both as a means of identifying its structure and hierarchies, and as a way of highlighting values inherent to the profession of nursing. Throughout the chapter, we will explore concepts and contexts that are relevant to developing your professional identity as both a nursing student and a registered nurse.

Developing a professional identity

In this section, we address concepts relevant to developing a professional identity as a registered nurse. The importance of self-awareness is explored as a foundation for effective reflective practice. Each of these domains is important for establishing effective strategies for communicating as a registered nurse.

Self-awareness

The concept of self-awareness is strongly linked to safe and effective nursing practice, largely because it is strongly associated with effective communication skills. Studies have linked heightened self-awareness in nurses to enhanced cultural **competence** (Caffrey et al., 2005), effective clinical communication strategies (Sheldon, Barrett & Ellington, 2006), student performance (Halfer & Graf, 2006), reflective practice (Gustafsson, Asp & Fagerberg, 2007) and effective leadership strategies (Horton-Deutsch & Sherwood, 2008). As a means of developing your professional identity, we will address your motivations for becoming a nurse in concert with your defining characteristics as an individual.

> **competence:**
> the ability to consistently function safely and effectively as a registered nurse

Motivations for becoming a nurse

As you embark on your career, you will probably be asked, 'Why did you choose nursing?' There is no right or wrong answer, as each individual will answer on the basis of their own perspective. Nursing may be something you chose out of genuine interest, for practical reasons or as a default option (Jirwe & Rudman, 2012). However, the reasons for your decision to pursue nursing studies and your level of motivation can have a significant effect on educational and professional outcomes because one day you may ask yourself, 'Why *did* I choose nursing?' Having a strong awareness of *why* you chose nursing – or why nursing chose you – is vital to your early and ongoing career development. You may wish to work in a tertiary referral hospital as part of a metropolitan trauma centre. Alternatively, you may be intrigued by the rigours and demands of rural and remote healthcare. Some students enter nursing with a view to caring for people in developing countries under the sponsorship of aid agencies or the military. However, not all students will enter nursing with such clear goals or ambitions beyond a simple desire to care for people in need.

By understanding your motivations for pursuing a career in nursing, you will begin to develop self-awareness. For instance, a 2008 study of pre-registration student nurses found that those with stronger self-efficacy (the strength of one's own awareness and ability to complete tasks and realise goals) were less likely to withdraw from their studies in nursing and more likely to perform at higher levels in their studies (McLaughlin, Moutray & Muldoon, 2008). Furthermore,

emotional intelligence – inclusive of self-awareness and motivation – was identified as having a potential impact on student learning, ethical decision-making, critical thinking, and the synthesis and integration of evidence in nursing practice (Bulmer Smith, Profetto-McGrath & Cummings, 2009). It is therefore very important to identify:

> **emotional intelligence:**
> the emotional and social characteristics, skills and enablers that determine how we perceive and express ourselves, understand and relate to others, and cope with daily living

- the factors that resulted in your current enrolment in a program of nursing education
- the personal characteristics that will inform your progression in scholarly and clinical environments, and
- your awareness of how the context that characterises your present circumstances will impact on your development as a safe and competent nurse.

Case study

You are your own case study for this exercise. Reflect honestly on what motivated you to become a nursing student, identifying at least three reasons.

Communicating your self-awareness

Not all students are enrolled in nursing because it is their ambition to become a registered nurse. Some students view nursing as a stepping-stone to a different profession. Some see it as a secondary choice: 'I had to do something so I chose nursing.' For some, nursing is something they will do for a while before they move on to 'something else'.

Not everyone will enter nursing because it 'called them'. Not everyone will have a story of a sick relative or friend whose illness ignited a caring flame in them that cannot be doused. Not everyone will see the opportunities that a career in nursing can offer individuals. However, everyone – at some point in their lives – will need a nurse.

Stop and think

Does this describe you? Historically, nursing was seen as a calling, which arguably implied that those who became nurses were automatically predisposed with qualities that would elicit consummate professionalism and profound compassion.

Critical reflection

>> What characteristics do you have that will enhance the benefit you derive from your learning experience?

>> What traits do you have that will make you a great nurse?

As you develop an awareness of yourself through carefully answering these questions, reflect on how your personal attributes will frame your learning experience, colour your nursing practice and shape the progression of your career in healthcare.

Becoming aware of your 'self'

Each individual possesses unique characteristics that impact positively – and sometimes negatively – on how they can contribute to nursing. For instance, you may have entered nursing with a deep desire to care for people, yet struggle with blood or needle phobias. You may be attracted to the high-pressure environments of the intensive care unit, the operating theatre or the emergency room, or you may be drawn to areas where you can build a unique rapport over time with patients and their families in aged care, rehabilitation or respite settings. Your motivation to work in these environments speaks as much about your individual characteristics as it does about the unique nature of care environments across the healthcare sector.

Having a strong sense of self-awareness is integral to developing ideas about your inherent strengths and weaknesses as a professional, as well as where and how you can best contribute as a registered nurse in the healthcare sector. A growing body of research around emotional intelligence in nursing has highlighted the need for nurses to possess emotional intelligence. As mentioned above, emotional intelligence is defined as the emotional and social characteristics, skills and enablers that determine how we perceive and express ourselves, understand others, relate to them and cope with daily living (Bar-On, 2005). Emotional intelligence is recognised as having an impact on the quality of student learning, ethical decision-making, critical thinking, evidence and knowledge use in practice, and patient outcomes (Bulmer Smith, Profetto-McGrath & Cummings, 2009). Furthermore, emotional intelligence can affect individuals' work outputs, general well-being and communication strategies (Salovey & Grewal, 2005). It impacts on a person's effectiveness in teams, their ability to recognise and respond appropriately to the feelings of self and others and their ability to encourage themselves and others (Cadman & Brewer, 2001).

An important early work by Goleman (2001) articulates the attributes or elements of emotional intelligence as follows:

- self-awareness (emotional awareness, esteem, insight)
- self-management (integrity, impulse control, adaptability)
- social awareness (developing others, managing conflict, bonding)
- relationship management (leadership, followership, work).

Although these attributes are not acquired quickly or easily, Clarke (2006) suggests that professional engagement and exposure to the healthcare environment facilitates the learning of emotional intelligence. For example, when caring for acutely ill patients, emotional intelligence is necessary to develop a nurse's self-awareness and to respond to the needs of the patient. This is done by the nurse acknowledging their own personal experience and perspective to discern an appropriate response, and identifying the strengths and weaknesses of the response to improve their practice. In the same context, self-management acknowledges the adaptability and capacity for control of nurses to deal with the changing pace and complex demands of the healthcare system. For instance, sudden alterations in a patient's condition will require a response that is appropriate to the needs of the patient and to the changing contexts of care. Social awareness in the nurse will be demonstrated by an ability to understand the emotional and social stressors caused by these sudden changes, and to work with the patient and their loved ones to achieve the best possible outcome.

professional identity: how an individual perceives and employs the characteristics that define their professional self

Finally, relationship management relates to the nurse's ability to work through the difficulties of the context – such as conflict, upheaval and change – and extract the best from people in order to instil confidence, trust and acceptance in others. These attributes will facilitate the development of your **professional identity** and stimulate your learning of emotional intelligence.

Having addressed the individual elements of how you define yourself and your professional identity, it is now appropriate to explore the broader context in which you will work, as a means of developing professional awareness.

Developing professional awareness

Developing a strong sense of self-awareness is vitally important to understanding the nursing profession and *how* it 'works'. Modern nursing is situated in a rapidly changing higher education and healthcare environment, with established systems designed to define and regulate the nursing profession. While the systematisation of nursing has existed in variety of forms for almost as long as the profession itself, in more recent times the roles, responsibilities and scopes of practice inherent to clinicians in the healthcare sector have been associated intrinsically with regulations, policies, practices and evidence. These elements within the system are designed to set forth the expected level of safe and effective practice that the system expects of nursing graduates.

You are a small yet significant cog in the wheel of this system; however, health professionals and health consumers share a very special interest in the safety and efficacy of graduating practitioners. This means your learning and professional progression are of great interest to the broader community – including the nursing profession. The progressive systematisation of nursing and healthcare is evidence of a concerted attempt to communicate to students, the profession and the public that you, as an individual, have a tremendous ability to make a difference in the system of which you are now a part. Identifying *how* you can make a difference – both in positive and negative terms – stems from a strong sense of professional identity and professional awareness. Comprehending the complexities of your professional role and responsibilities, both as a nursing student and registered nurse, will further enable you to understand not only what the system expects of you, but what you should expect of yourself. Exploring both these perspectives during your progression towards beginning nursing practice will help you to form an appropriate response to the requirements of registered nursing practice. In the next section, we explore the roles of the nursing student and the registered nurse.

The roles of the nursing student and the healthcare professional

Your level of motivation will also play a significant role in how you receive and respond to the communicated expectations articulated by the system. Whether private or public, metropolitan, or rural and remote, healthcare systems are fallible; however, the nursing profession has established frameworks to promote the safety and efficacy of nurses through the use of legislation, professional requirements, codes, **accreditation** and competency frameworks (Birks, Chapman & Ralph, 2014).

> **accreditation:**
> a process by which an assessing entity (for example, a professional body) evaluates the credibility, reliability and validity of a program (such as an educational program) presented by another party for the purposes of approving its fitness for purpose

The structural organisation of both the higher education and healthcare systems communicates clearly to nursing students and nurses alike that a high standard of professionalism is expected of them. Since the inception of the Australian Health Practitioners Regulation Agency (AHPRA), all students enrolled in an approved program of study in nursing or those who are undertaking clinical training in nursing have been mandatorily registered with the Nursing and Midwifery Board of Australia (NMBA) (NMBA, 2014). For the same reasons that health practitioners are registered, nursing students are also listed with the NMBA to protect public safety and allow for appropriate steps to be taken when a serious contravention of the conditions of a student's registration (such as evidence of an impairment or serious misconduct) has occurred (AHPRA, 2014).

Such stringent requirements may come as a surprise to nursing students. However, the intent of this chapter is to highlight the system-wide communications that are geared towards the high standards established for nursing students and nurses who operate within the higher education and healthcare sectors.

Person-centredness

The systems of higher education and healthcare are multifaceted and extraordinarily complex. It is important to remember that the intent of these highly structured systems is to facilitate approaches to education and healthcare delivery that primarily benefit the individual in need of care. Such an approach translates to the concept of patient or person-centredness as a guiding ethos in both the preparation of nursing students for professional practice and the practice of registered nurses working in the clinical setting.

Person-centredness was initially articulated as an approach and a standard of care that prioritise the patient/client at the centre of care delivery (McCormack, Manley & Titchen, 2013). In order to explain the concept more clearly, we will examine the principle of person-centredness and its influence on healthcare and education.

Healthcare

As a current or future healthcare professional, you will communicate almost constantly in ways unique to the contexts of healthcare. For instance, communication between health professionals often occurs in an extremely structured way, using pre-determined and agreed-upon frameworks. In one moment, you may communicate through structured handovers using mnemonics such as ISOBAR (Identify, Situation, Observations, Background, Agreed Plan, Read Back), or perhaps frameworks of documented communication such as SOAP (Subjective, Objective, Assessment, Plan). Whatever the case, such a structure reflects the expectation that clarity, accuracy and detail are the hallmarks of communication between health professionals.

Often occurring simultaneously with *structured* communication is the *unstructured* communication that occurs between the patient or their loved ones and the practitioner. Strong and effective communication between the patient and the practitioner is the cornerstone of safe and effective therapeutic relationships. The need for trust, respect and rapport – often in times of great difficulty and distress in a person's life – is vital to mitigating the discomfort that periods of illness can impose on people's lives. In many senses, healthcare is unique in the almost instantaneous changes it demands of those who are responsible for the delivery of care. In one sense, communicating through the extreme structure of clinical handover and documentation is often simultaneously juxtaposed with the unpredictable and complex contexts brought to bear by persons requiring a nursing presence.

It is arguably the concept of the nursing presence that distinguishes nurses from all other healthcare professionals. Nurses are far more present than other healthcare practitioners, and consequently are placed in a privileged position to be able to constantly assess, observe and act on changes to the needs of the patient. Therefore, in terms of the nursing profession, the concept of person-centredness comes from the fact that nursing has *always* valued the privilege of presence in that it enables nurses to provide a person-centred experience throughout care. Nurses will adapt to the needs of the person using communication – whether that need is to communicate the patient's condition to colleagues through clear and accurate documentation or handover, or to reassure the patient with whom the nurse has built a strong therapeutic relationship by using their expert communication skills.

Education

In the higher education sector, much is made of the student experience. The importance of providing each student with a rich experience at university is often recognised by the extensive support systems, social clubs, facilities and events that characterise university life. These initiatives are intended to provide a supportive environment to students, which facilitates a rich and relevant learning experience for each individual.

In nursing education, the most appropriate way to provide a valuable student experience is to diffuse person-centred approaches through the strategies used to facilitate learning and teaching. As addressed throughout this chapter, the purpose of each system – whether healthcare or higher education – is to ensure that each graduate who completes a program of formal education is safe, competent and relevant to the needs of the Australian healthcare consumer.

In this respect, your ability to articulate an awareness of yourself and the factors that motivated you towards a career in health is very important if you

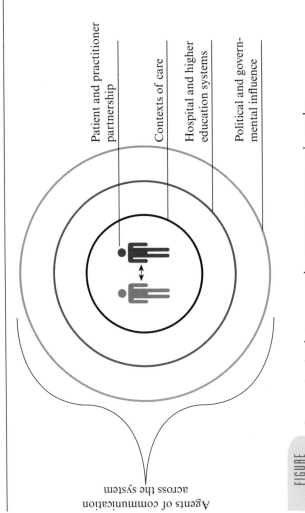

Patient and practitioner
partnership

Contexts of care

Hospital and higher
education systems

Political and govern-
mental influence

Agents of communication
across the system

FIGURE
1.1

Communication between people, contexts, systems and agendas

are to interpret how *you* can use what you bring to the profession in ways that benefit the person in need of healthcare.

Throughout both systems, using person-centredness to guide the delivery of healthcare and to facilitate learning in nursing education is common. In higher education, the focus on curriculum is indisputably professed to be person-centred. The preparation of health practitioners is almost exclusively focused on educating students of nursing and other health disciplines towards optimising their capacity to provide safe and competent care to those in need.

Across the healthcare system, one fact is clearly communicated: that the position of the patient or person is at the epicentre of all activities. These two systems work in tandem to articulate to the profession, the public and the person that the needs of the individual requiring care must be prioritised. The importance of the partnership between practitioner and person is therefore paramount, and a strong, therapeutic, person-centred relationship between the caregiver and care receiver is fundamental to realising the very existential purpose of each of these systems (see Figure 1.1).

In explaining this partnership, you will no doubt be confronted by one of the nuances of communication: the almost mutually interchangeable terms of 'patient' and 'client'. While some traditionalists might argue for the term 'patient', its roots are derived from the Latin *patiens*, meaning 'to suffer' (Baruch, 2010). More recently, the term 'client' has risen in use throughout nursing and healthcare to denote the transaction that occurs in healthcare between the person and the practitioner. In many respects, the word 'client' is arguably a means of communicating that the partnership between the person being cared for and the care-providing practitioner involves mutual expectations that bring certain rights and responsibilities for both parties. The guiding values and responsibilities of the nurse in this partnership are clearly articulated in the *Code of Professional Conduct for Nurses in Australia* (NMBA, 2008b) and *Code of Ethics for Nurses in Australia* (NMBA, 2008a) and provide a pathway to how professional practice must be constantly conducted in all contexts of care.

Pathways to professional practice

While there may be many different pathways to an individual undertaking studies in nursing or pursuing a career in healthcare, the pathways to professional practice are reflective of a more structured environment, due to the need for a system that prepares people to become safe, effective and relevant practitioners who can meet the broader needs of the health-consuming public.

Guiding lights in the nursing profession

The nursing profession in Australia is guided by many documents that provide codes, guidelines and policies for the good of nurses across the country.

Codes of practice

Two of the most significant documents relating to the essence of nursing are:

- the *Code of Ethics for Nurses in Australia* (NMBA, 2008a), and
- the *Code of Professional Conduct for Nurses in Australia* (NMBA, 2008b).

The *Code of Ethics for Nurses in Australia* was developed for the Australian nursing profession using key documents from the United Nations and the World Health Organization to inform its conceptualisation. The code is clearly designed to communicate the ethical or moral values nurses are expected to uphold to a broad audience, from nurses to nursing students, employers, organisations, regulatory authorities, the broader community and health consumers. Broadly speaking, there are eight value statements, which are outlined in greater detail within the *Code of Ethics for Nurses in Australia* (see box).

Code of Ethics for Nurses in Australia

1. Nurses value quality nursing care for all people.
2. Nurses value respect and kindness for self and others.
3. Nurses value the diversity of people.
4. Nurses value access to quality nursing and healthcare for all people.
5. Nurses value informed decision-making.
6. Nurses value a culture of safety in nursing and healthcare.
7. Nurses value ethical management of information.
8. Nurses value a socially, economically and ecologically sustainable environment promoting health and wellbeing. (NMBA, 2008a)

Through these statements, the professional commitment of nursing is to respect, promote, protect and uphold the human rights of people receiving care and the nurses providing it. The values articulated by the *Code of Ethics for Nurses in Australia* underpin the *Code of Professional Conduct for Nurses in*

Australia (see box) which refers to the behaviours expected of a nurse relevant to their professional role.

Code of Professional Conduct for Nurses in Australia

1 Nurses practise in a safe and competent manner.

2 Nurses practise in accordance with the standards of the profession and broader health system.

3 Nurses practise and conduct themselves in accordance with laws relevant to the profession and practice of nursing.

4 Nurses respect the dignity, culture, ethnicity, values and beliefs of people receiving care and treatment, and of their colleagues.

5 Nurses treat personal information obtained in a professional capacity as private and confidential.

6 Nurses provide impartial, honest and accurate information in relation to nursing care and healthcare products.

7 Nurses support the health, wellbeing and informed decision-making of people requiring or receiving care.

8 Nurses promote and preserve the trust and privilege inherent in the relationship between nurses and people receiving care.

9 Nurses maintain and build on the community's trust and confidence in the nursing profession.

10 Nurses practise nursing reflectively and ethically. (NMBA, 2008b)

Interestingly, both codes are binding, whether within or outside the professional domain of practice. In essence, nurses are expected to be of good standing within the profession and also within the community (NMBA, 2008a). The moment you enrolled in a nursing program, you became subject to the values espoused by the nursing profession and the standards of professional conduct required by its members.

Accreditation standards

In 2010, the National Registration and Accreditation Scheme (NRAS) came into effect, and with it the birth of the Australian Nursing and Midwifery Accreditation Council (ANMAC). For the first time in Australian history, programs of nursing and midwifery education were accredited according to the same standards across the nation. Previously, state- and territory-based accreditation bodies employed different standards to accredit programs that led to registration as a nurse or a midwife. Historically, the differences in state and territory approaches to accreditation resulted in significant variations in both the quality and focus of education in the disciplines of nursing and midwifery (Ralph, Birks & Chapman, 2015).

ANMAC plays a significant role in ensuring the health and safety of the Australian health consumer by facilitating a high standard of nursing and midwifery education (ANMAC, 2015). Together with the Nursing and Midwifery Board of Australia (NMBA), ANMAC works as a regulatory partner to:

- establish, revise and develop standards of accreditation for nursing and midwifery programs
- accredit Australian nursing and midwifery education providers and the programs they deliver, leading to a qualification that includes registration or endorsement as a nurse
- develop, review and provide policy advice and skills assessments of nurses and midwives with international qualifications, who apply to migrate and work in Australia.

As a result of its scope of service, ANMAC provides a vital role in promoting public safety by regulating the education and health sectors to ensure that only health practitioners who are appropriately trained, educated or qualified to practise in a competent and ethical manner are eligible for registration in Australia. While AHPRA regulates the registration status of individual health practitioners across the nation, it is ANMAC, in concert with the NMBA, that is instrumental in ensuring only those who have undertaken appropriate pathways to registration or endorsement as a nurse or midwife are eligible for registration. Under the auspices of its role in accrediting more than 400 programs of education across more than 160 providers of education, ANMAC partners with nursing education to embed a standard of quality by enforcing accreditation standards (Ralph, Birks & Chapman, 2013). Through its role, ANMAC ensures each program can produce graduates of a standard conducive to the continued quality and safety of both the Australian nursing profession and the healthcare sector.

Throughout this system, the messages being sent are clear: Australian health consumers expect graduates to be educated to a high standard, ready to practise at a pre-defined level, and able to function in a safe and competent manner. The system of accreditation is another example of a system hard-wired to communicate a standard of educational progression in keeping with the standards set forth by the nursing profession in Australia. Accreditation standards communicate to the education provider, the profession, the students and the health consumer that high standards are expected across the system,

TABLE 1.1 *Summary of domains in the National Competency Standards for the Registered Nurse*

DOMAIN	EXPLANATION
Professional practice	This relates to the professional, legal and ethical responsibilities that require demonstration of a satisfactory knowledge base, accountability for practice, functioning in accordance with legislation affecting nursing and healthcare, and the protection of individual and group rights.
Critical thinking and analysis	This relates to self-appraisal, professional development and the value of evidence and research for practice. Reflecting on practice, feelings and beliefs, and the consequences of these for individuals/groups, is an important professional benchmark.
Provision and coordination of care	This domain relates to the coordination, organisation and provision of nursing care that includes the assessment of individuals/groups, planning, implementation and evaluation of care.
Collaborative and therapeutic practice	This relates to establishing, sustaining and concluding professional relationships with individuals/groups. It also contains those competencies that relate to nurses' understanding of their contribution to the interdisciplinary healthcare team.

Source: NMBA (2008c)

to ensure those applying to become registered health practitioners are safe and competent to use their relevant skills and knowledge to improve healthcare delivery across Australia.

Communicating learning objectives and outcomes

One of the pivotal issues for anyone enrolled in pre-registration nursing programs is the question of what they are meant to learn and the outcomes of their learning. For students in nursing, the *National Competency Standards for the Registered Nurse* (NMBA, 2008c) are the key outcomes of their learning on completing their education program. The *National Competency Standards* are used to identify the requisite level of performance expected of registered nurses to obtain and retain registration in Australia. They also inform the standards of accreditation in Australia, thereby influencing not only the standards of practice of nurses but also the intent and focus of pre-registration nursing programs in the country. It is useful as you progress towards the completion of your education to reflect on how your learning has developed your competency in the four domains of competency standards in nursing (see Table 1.1).

The competency standards are communicating the required standard of clinical performance expected from you as well as every other individual registered or registering as a nurse in Australia. Whereas the *Code of Ethics for Nurses in Australia* and the *Code of Professional Conduct for Nurses in Australia* articulate both the values and behaviours that will guide and characterise the nursing profession, the *National Competency Standards for the Registered Nurse in Australia* communicate the expected standards of clinical performance, irrespective of the specialisations, experiences or qualifications of nurses across the nation. As you progress through your course, be sure to familiarise yourself with the learning objectives of each subject you undertake and the overall program objectives. Use them to not only understand what you *need* to learn and what is *expected* of you, but also to reflect on what you *have* learned. This exercise will provide you with useful information to identify the strengths and weakness of your learning experience and will help you to articulate to potential employers how you have progressed from a first-year student to a safe, competent and relevant graduate who will bring highly employable skills, knowledge and qualities to the healthcare environment.

Summary

In establishing the contexts of communication, it is important to develop both a sense of professional identity through learned emotional intelligence and a broad professional awareness. Having an understanding of both of these areas is key to identifying your roles, responsibilities and potential contributions to the profession of nursing and to patients. By gaining insight into yourself and the profession of which you are now a part, you will be able to approach the information contained in subsequent chapters of the textbook with a greater appreciation of how to effectively communicate in your role as a care provider.

Discussion and critical thinking questions

1.1 What strengths and abilities do you possess that will enable you to work professionally in new learning and professional nursing contexts?

1.2 Provide some examples of your professional approach in your role as a student and on clinical practice.

1.3 Describe the patient-centred framework.

1.4 What are professional requirements/pathways to professional nursing practice?

1.5 What are some of the forces of change operating in the healthcare context?

Learning extension

In this chapter, you considered your motivation for undertaking nursing studies. How does this motivation, or the reasons you gave for wanting to start a nursing career, intersect with the need for professionalism in your roles as a student and nurse? What is your understanding of professionalism? What strategies will you incorporate into your modus operandi to reflect on and build your capacity to be professional in your practices as a student and as a nurse?

References

Arnold, E.C. & Boggs, K.U. (2013). *Interpersonal relationships: Professional communication skills for nurses.* New York: Elsevier.

Australian Health Practitioners Regulation Agency (AHPRA) (2014). FAQ for education providers. Retrieved 14 August 2014 from <http://www.ahpra.gov.au/ Registration/Student-Registrations/FAQ-for-Education-Providers.aspx>.

Australian Nursing and Midwifery Accreditation Council (ANMAC) (2015). Website. Retrieved 20 January 2015 from <http://www.anmac.org.au>.

Bar-On, R. (2005). The impact of emotional intelligence on subjective well-being. *Perspectives in Education,* 23(2): 1–22.

Baruch, J. (2010). Gaps in the safety net metaphor. *Virtual Mentor,* 12(6): 487–91.

Birks, M., Chapman, Y. & Ralph, N. (2014). Assisting the transition: Establishment of a first year experience coordinator role for nursing students. *New Developments in Nursing Education Research.* New York: Nova Science.

Bulmer Smith, K., Profetto-McGrath, J. & Cummings, G.G. (2009). Emotional intelligence and nursing: An integrative literature review. *International Journal of Nursing Studies,* 46(12): 1624–36.

Cadman, C. & Brewer, J. (2001). Emotional intelligence: A vital prerequisite for recruitment in nursing. *Journal of Nursing Management,* 9(6): 321–4.

Caffrey, R.A., Neander, W., Markle, D. & Stewart, B. (2005). Improving the cultural competence of nursing students: Results of integrating cultural content in the curriculum and an international immersion experience. *The Journal of Nursing Education,* 44(5): 234–40.

Clarke, N. (2006). Developing emotional intelligence through workplace learning: Findings from a case study in healthcare. *Human Resource Development International,* 9(4): 447–65.

Goleman, D. (2001). An EI-based theory of performance. In C. Cherniss & D. Goleman (eds), *The emotionally intelligent workplace: How to select for, measure, and improve emotional intelligence in individuals, groups, and organizations.* New York: Jossey-Bass.

Gustafsson, C., Asp, M. & Fagerberg, I. (2007). Reflective practice in nursing care: Embedded assumptions in qualitative studies. *International Journal of Nursing Practice*, 13(3): 151–60.

Halfer, D. & Graf, E. (2006). Graduate nurse perceptions of the work experience. *Nursing Economics*, 24(3): 150–5.

Haynes, A.B., Weiser, T.G., Berry, W.R., Lipsitz, S.R., Breizat, A.H.S., Dellinger, E.P., Dziekan, G. & Gawande, A.A. (2011). Changes in safety attitude and relationship to decreased postoperative morbidity and mortality following implementation of a checklist-based surgical safety intervention. *BMJ Quality & Safety*, 20(1): 102–7.

Horton-Deutsch, S. & Sherwood, G. (2008). Reflection: An educational strategy to develop emotionally competent nurse leaders. *Journal of Nursing Management*, 16(8): 946–54.

Hughes, R. & Mitchell, P. (2008). Defining patient safety and quality care. In R. Hughes (ed.), *Patient safety and quality: An evidence-based handbook for nurses*. Rockville, MD: AHRQ.

Jirwe, M. & Rudman, A. (2012). Why choose a career in nursing? *Journal of Advanced Nursing*, 68(7): 1615–23.

Kernbach, S., Eppler, M.J. & Bresciani, S. (2014). The use of visualization in the communication of business strategies: An experimental evaluation. *International Journal of Business Communication*, doi: 10.1177/2329488414525444.

Leonard, M., Graham, S. & Bonacum, D. (2004). The human factor: The critical importance of effective teamwork and communication in providing safe care. *Quality and Safety in Health Care*, 13(Suppl. 1): i85–i90.

Lin, E.C.L., Chen, S.L., Chao, S.Y. & Chen, Y.C. (2013). Using standardized patient with immediate feedback and group discussion to teach interpersonal and communication skills to advanced practice nursing students. *Nurse Education Today*, 33(6): 677–83.

McCormack, B., Manley, K. & Titchen, A. (eds) (2013). *Practice development in nursing and healthcare*. Hoboken, NJ: John Wiley & Sons.

McLaughlin, K., Moutray, M. & Muldoon, O.T. (2008). The role of personality and self-efficacy in the selection and retention of successful nursing students: A longitudinal study. *Journal of Advanced Nursing*, 61(2): 211–21.

Mills, P., Neily, J. & Dunn, E. (2008). Teamwork and communication in surgical teams: Implications for patient safety. *Journal of the American College of Surgeons*, 206(1): 107–12.

Nursing and Midwifery Board of Australia (NMBA) (2008a). *Code of Ethics for Nurses in Australia*. Canberra: NMBA.

—— (2008b). *Code of Professional Conduct for Nurses in Australia*. Canberra: NMBA.

—— (2008c). *National Competency Standards for the Registered Nurse*. Canberra: NMBA.

—— (2014). Student registration. Retrieved 14 August 2014, from <http://www.
nursingmidwiferyboard.gov.au/Registration-and-Endorsement/Student-
Registration.aspx>.

Ralph, N., Birks, M. & Chapman, Y. (2015). The accreditation of nursing education in
Australia. *Collegian*, 22(1): 3–7.

Salovey, P. & Grewal, D. (2005). The science of emotional intelligence. *Current
Directions in Psychological Science*, 14(6): 281–5.

Sheldon, L.K., Barrett, R. & Ellington, L. (2006). Difficult communication in nursing.
Journal of Nursing Scholarship, 38(2): 141–7.

Veil, S.R., Buehner, T. & Palenchar, M.J. (2011). A work-in-process literature
review: Incorporating social media in risk and crisis communication. *Journal of
Contingencies and Crisis Management*, 19(2): 110–22.

2 Communication theory and its applications in nursing and healthcare

Eleanor Kiernan

Learning objectives

- Recognise that theory is the initial stage of problem-solving that can have real-life applications and improve as theories are tested.

- Have an understanding of three models of communication that have evolved to better explain the complexities of communication.

- Apply elements of the transactional model – particularly barriers and strategies – to the nursing context.

- Develop insights into communication behaviours that could negatively affect colleagues and patients.

Key terms

- Code

- Communication models

- Context

- Empathy

- Interpersonal barriers

- Intrapersonal/psychological barriers

- Noise

- Physical barriers

- Semantic barriers

- Validation

Introduction

Nursing students sometimes get impatient with ideas that are not practice-based. Because they are busy people, they are often more interested in learning content or gaining clinical nursing knowledge to equip them for their professional lives. Some nursing students may consider that learning about communication theory is irrelevant, as they feel that communication is something that can be taken for granted and therefore does not need special attention. However, this is a short-sighted view, as understanding the dynamics of communication can help students by providing opportunities to look at challenging communication incidents through a more analytical and objective prism. Of course, there is no single blueprint for successful communication, as there are so many variables that can affect the communication process. At the very least, though, communication theory can help give the nursing student some perspective and provide a springboard for analysis and possible solutions to a problem. Nursing students will eventually come to have a deep understanding of the causes and effects of illness and changes in the human body, and investigate the theories and research related to them. This chapter argues that a similar approach should be taken to communication. Using the transactional model of communication as a catalyst for discussion, the chapter explores elements that relate to effective communication, including communication barriers, strategies, channels and context, to investigate how it can be applied in nursing. Perception, which underpins all communication, will be considered to show how people's world-views are unique, which in turn makes each communication episode ripe with opportunities but susceptible to potential risks.

Rationale for the development of theory

Nursing students normally have a very heavy workload, as their studies include a great deal of complexity and intellectual rigour to adequately prepare them for their nursing careers. Given the time pressures these demands place on students, they may want to concentrate on the clinical nursing subjects or areas that they perceive to be more relevant and specific to nursing. Understanding communication theory therefore may not appear to be a high priority – indeed, it may seem redundant, as most people think they know how to communicate. Unfortunately, such thinking may lead to lost opportunities, as an understanding of the many dimensions of the human being, including the physical and the psychological elements that fuel human communication, can help extend the nurse's understanding and repertoire of skills in interpersonal communication. Effective communication is vital at all levels of nursing, and understanding the theory and the dynamics behind communication can help to improve emotional intelligence (see Chapters 1 and 8), which in turn will improve nursing practice.

Communication theory

Theory is a system of applying a series of ideas or possibilities in a systematic way to try to explain a phenomenon or solve a problem. Griffin (2009, pp. 4–5) explains it more fully:

> A theory not only lays out multiple ideas, but also specifies relationships among them. In common parlance, it connects the dots. The links among the informed hunches are clearly drawn so that a whole pattern emerges.

Although we do not always realise it, we often develop theories as a means of explaining aspects of our lives and environment. For example, as a nurse you may notice that a long-term patient is always rude and obnoxious to the staff after his visitors leave. As the patient is normally pleasant, you may theorise after repeated observations of this behaviour that the patient feels lonely and isolated once his family has gone. You could extrapolate from this inductive evidence to make a broader conclusion that visitors can upset a patient's equilibrium, and this can cause short-term distress. In this situation, you have mentally developed a theory and have a basis for understanding similar situations. The theory may or may not collapse if explored in a rigorous way, but you have nonetheless developed a theory – albeit perhaps unwittingly.

Communication models

In this chapter, we will 'connect the dots' by looking at how communication works, based on evolving descriptions of the communication process.

communication models: ways of describing communication in a diagrammatic form; for example, the linear, interactive and transaction models

Communication models are a useful way of seeing how a theory can be represented in a diagrammatic form, which can help to show the relationships as stated in Griffin's definition of theory.

Communication models have evolved from the first rudimentary model by Shannon and Weaver in 1949, which described transmission. This linear model was fairly mechanistic, and basically reflected the idea that the sender and receiver had little to do with the interpretation of the message, which was essentially independent. However, if this were true, every time you went to a lecture, you would be able to understand the many messages conveyed to you without any explanation. Of course, the reality is that if you're tired, distracted, overwhelmed and uncertain, the message will not be received in the way it was intended. This model also did not reflect the two-way nature of communication. It did, however, introduce the concept of the communication barrier – although only to a limited extent. It included *physical noise*, which meant anything that interfered with the transmission of a message, such as static on the radio line or your computer crashing.

Clearly, there are problems with the linear model in explaining how communication works, and better models evolved to better represent communication. Nonetheless, the linear model was useful as a critical starting point, and it helped to establish some common terms that have been adapted into other models, including:

- sender/receiver – source and destination
- message – the information being conveyed
- **code** – the system used to convey the information, words, graphs, non-verbal communication, etc.
- channel – the way the code is conveyed – for example, it may be easier to present complex information in a graph rather than by using the written word
- **noise** – communication barrier.

> **code:** a set of symbols that are combined to build a communication message – for example, type of language or graphic representations
>
> **noise:** a communication theory term – any barrier that affects the transmission of a message

As a nursing student, you may already have thought about the code or channel you use when communicating. For example, a patient may not be able to hear well, so you may have to write out the message. Emailing lecturers rather than seeing them face to face may be a choice based on your mode of study, convenience or anxiety, but one that you hope will achieve the best results. You will also need to consider non-verbal communication, as it makes up a significant proportion of communication (see Chapter 6). In the healthcare space, some patients may have to rely on non-verbal communication, depending on their condition. So, when communicating, you need to choose the channel and the code that are most effective at the time.

Thus, while there are some aspects of the linear model that represent what actually happens when we communicate (for example, the code or channel), the linear model does not reflect enough of the elements that describe communication. Unfortunately, some people communicate as if the linear model were accurate. For example, have you been to a lecture where the lecturers don't ask for questions or take advantage of feedback? It is almost as though they believe

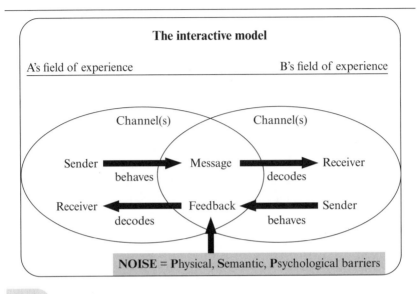

The interactive model of communication

they just need to deliver information and that you will receive it in the way it was meant with 100 per cent accuracy. This impedes meaningful and efficient communication.

The *interactive model of communication* (see Figure 2.1) is an advance on the linear model, as it reflects the communicator's fields of experience (see below). It also includes more barriers – semantic, psychological and interpersonal. Most importantly, it includes two-way feedback, so it accurately represents what happens when we communicate. The initial impression is that this model provides a clearer explanation of how communication works. It introduces significant improvements: the two-way process and the field of experience. The number of barriers is expanded to include psychological and semantic barriers. However, the main problem is that it looks at communication as if it were tidy and predictable. It suggests that communication happens in discrete stages. 'A' asks a question of 'B', who then replies and the process is repeated. Unfortunately, this does not reflect the reality of communication, as the way people talk is often messy. They interrupt and talk at the same time, which can make it less of a 'clean' process. It could, however, be used to describe communication that does occur in discrete chunks, such as emails, forum discussions, Facebook messages and even (rare now) letters.

The *transactional model of communication* (see Figure 2.2) added some important additional elements: the simultaneous and continuous nature of communication. It also added the interpersonal barrier, which is fundamental to human communication. Communication strategies are also included, which closes off the communication process (see below for a more in-depth discussion on communication barriers and strategies). The field of experience is what people bring to the communication experience, as we do not communicate in a vacuum. It is basically the individual, cultural, psychological and environmental variables that have created the way the person sees the world – these include factors such as values, sex, age, occupation, education, financial status, mood, memory, family background and personal relationships, to name a few. This field of experience shapes the way we perceive the message and ultimately our world-view. Chapters 3, 4 and 5 also discuss perception or world-view and its influence on communication.

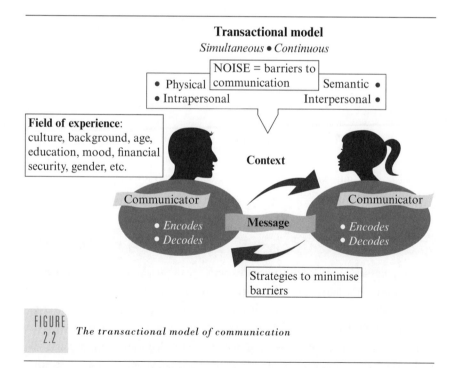

FIGURE 2.2 *The transactional model of communication*

People's unique world-views: Perception

As we go through each day, we need some kind of filtering system to help us process the constant assault on our senses by the multitude of stimuli in our environment. If we did not have such a filtering system, we would be exposed to so much information that we couldn't mentally cope with it. Therefore, we need to make sense of the world: this is our *perception*, which creates our world-view. Perception is 'the active process of creating meaning by selecting, organizing, and interpreting people, objects, events, situations, and other phenomena' (Wood, 2013). The field of experience mentioned in Figure 2.2 contributes to our perception, as do multiple layers of experience. We can have similar view-points to others, but there will always be slight variations because each person is unique.

Siblings have similar backgrounds but many variables will affect their perception, such as birth order, different experiences at school and so on. Our perception is not cemented and can change over time – even seemingly intractable beliefs and values can be shifted. Once stereotypes of people are broken down, people may have a more realistic understanding and therefore their perceptions can change. For example, Spiteri's (2013) study of school-boys showed that when the boys had contact and open dialogue with young asylum seekers about their traumas and difficulties, the boys' perceptions and prejudices were reduced and replaced with a more empathetic attitude. Chapter 5 examines the impact of perception in communication. In cross-cultural theory, perception is known as a 'cultural world-view' or 'way of knowing'.

context: the time, place and relationship of something, which can determine the meaning of communication

Our perception is affected by another important element of the transactional model: **context**. Time, place and relationship are important aspects of context, and can affect the success of the message.

Time

As time passes, you have different experiences that shape your perspective. As an undergraduate nursing student, your perceptions will change as you progress through your degree and gain knowledge and maturity, so your vision of the world will change. An example that shows how your world-view can change is your choice of career. You may have enrolled in nursing because you had certain perceptions of it. Highly dramatised television programs or other media can often shape these perceptions; students are sometimes attracted to nursing specialisations that are reflected in films and television as being exciting or glamorous, and this affects their initial choice (Birks et al., 2014). As some of the myths are dispelled and the reality is revealed, you will look at nursing in more sophisticated ways. Another aspect related to time is *when* the message takes place. Your timing can torpedo or enhance the success of the message. For example, as a nursing student, you may need an extension for an assignment, but contacting your lecturer at 5.00 p.m. on the day it is due may not be the most propitious time to ask for it. So time is a significant part of the complex communication process.

Place

Where the communication takes place will determine how well it is received. For example, talking about your weekend when you are involved in an emergency situation at the hospital may not be regarded as the ideal place for such a discussion.

Relationship

Our relationship with people helps to shape the way we perceive and interact with others. How intimate we are with people has an impact on our expectations. This also relates to our professional relationships. If a nursing student has a good relationship with some patients but not others, a negative attitude will be revealed to the problematic patients, no matter how hard the student tries to hide their true feelings. We betray ourselves by many of the different types of non-verbal communication, such as tone of voice (paralinguistics) and body language (kinesics) (see Chapter 6).

Communication barriers

Think about the following case study.

Case study

Mika (a first-year nursing student) explains how she tried to analyse her problems by using basic communication theory.

According to communication theory, my communication difficulties come from three major barriers. First, my communication issues with flatmates come from gender differences. As a woman, I am concerned about cleaning and noise, but my male flatmates don't care. This communication problem is an interpersonal barrier which can be created because of different values and perspectives. Second, physical barriers are created by loud music and parties, and this can also lead to problems with my flatmates, which then develop into another interpersonal barrier. As an international student, I am also aware of semantic barriers, as I sometimes don't have confidence in my English. This in turn creates psychological barriers because it creates anxiety.

Critical reflection

》 Reflect on the communication barriers Mika is experiencing. Write short notes about how you would solve these problems if you were Mika.

Mika is thinking carefully about her problems, and is applying aspects of the transactional model to them. This is a good example of how something that starts out as theory can have useful applications and be the starting point for problem-solving. As you progress through your studies and nursing career, you can be mindful and analytical about your communication. An understanding of intrapersonal, interpersonal, semantic and physical (or external) barriers can help to increase your emotional intelligence. It is worth noting that many of these barriers are sometimes interdependent and create overlap. For example, Mika's semantic barriers ended up creating an intrapersonal or psychological barrier: anxiety.

Intrapersonal/psychological barriers

As nursing students and future professionals, you will be confronted by many situations that will make you uneasy, where communication barriers have arisen between you and the people with whom you are communicating. Some of these situations can be based on:

- assumptions and expectations
- fear and anxiety
- stereotyping (leading to bias and prejudice) and labelling.

intrapersonal/ psychological barriers: barriers within a person, such as bias, anxiety and assumptions, that impede communication

Intrapersonal/psychological barriers can stem from assumptions and differing expectations. For example, nursing students can make assumptions about staff or patients, thus creating potential problems. A study of nursing students found that assumptions made about a patient's diet were challenged after astute questioning by a nursing student (Jirwe, Gerrish & Emami, 2010). The patient notes indicated that the patient would eat everything, and the nursing student reiterated this idea to the patient, who confirmed it was correct. However, the nursing student then asked the patient whether she ate pork, and the answer was no. This then led to a useful discussion where clearer information was given and both the patient and the nursing student were pleased with the result. This is an example of where a person did not accept an idea at face value. However, the same nursing student asked another patient (a man from an Islamic country) whether he ate pork (he didn't) and this unfortunately created offence because of assumptions about religious differences (Jirwe, Gerrish & Emami, 2010), which therefore led to interpersonal barriers. This example illustrates the challenges nursing students face, and reflects the idea that not everyone will respond in a predictable way. It also suggests nurses need to be psychologically robust to deal with the vagaries of nursing life, as confidence can be built and diminished in the same shift.

Physicians may have expectations and assumptions about nurses that can also create communication barriers within the team, with potential risks for all concerned. In a study of oncology nursing, Wittenberg-Lyles, Goldsmith and Ferrell (2013) found that doctors sometimes failed to give the full picture about patient care because they assumed and expected that the nurse would already have this knowledge. This can have a potentially dire effect on patient care, particularly in the highly sensitive end-of-life care context, and could negatively affect the new nurse's confidence when conveying observations that could be useful to the physician. Thus this circle of unresolved communication strands can create a poor communication climate because of these communication barriers.

Personal or political situations can generate fear and anxiety, which can also affect the nurse's perception of the patient and ultimately patient care. Nursing students may unconsciously (or even consciously) blame the patient for things beyond their control. A climate of fear can often create poor behaviour, even if it is subtle, and this can have a deleterious impact on the patient. For example, some commentators have noted that people of Middle Eastern origin around the world are subject to racism and prejudice in healthcare settings. Unfortunately, this type of issue has real consequences, and affects the health outcomes for patients and creates further psychological problems including lowered self-esteem, social withdrawal and increased marginalisation (Al Abed et al., 2014). Of course, this applies to many other groups in our society, and if nursing students are aware of the causes of prejudice and possible impacts on patient care, it could help to reduce their negative behaviour (even if it is not intentional).

This kind of behaviour could be linked to labelling theory. Price (2013) states that labelling theory relates to the practices that some people construct to disadvantage the less powerful in society. Price's discussion related to negative attitudes towards older people, who are sometimes perceived to be less productive and therefore less worthy of attention. If other groups are also labelled in a negative way, they can also be the victims of poor decision-making. Doctors and nurses are the gatekeepers and decision-makers for vital services and facilities, and intrapersonal barriers such as assumptions can lead to stereotyping, bias and even prejudice. This could unfairly disadvantage some patients and compromise patient care. Labelling theory is an example of a theory that can be applied to a specific context to help analyse a situation. Being aware of this theory, and taking steps to avoid these kinds of behaviours, can help overcome the intrapersonal barriers related to labelling and stereotyping.

Intrapersonal barriers are present in all human beings; they are part of our cultural and psychological history. Nursing students are no different from anyone else, but because your attitudes could potentially affect the way you treat colleagues and patients, it is important to develop emotional intelligence and take a 'stocktake' of these attitudes. As indicated throughout many chapters in this book, self-awareness is a critical starting point to changing perceptions and improving professionalism. Other strategies often stem from awareness, and particularly self-awareness.

Empathy

Empathy is trying to understand the other person's perspective, and it is a useful characteristic in human communication. If you really try to see the other person's position, it helps to create more meaningful conversation, which could result in more creative problem-solving. The starting point for developing empathy is *empathic listening*, which goes beyond merely comprehending the words and centres on really trying to understand the other person's situation, feelings or motives (Engleberg & Wynn, 2015). Empathic listening can help to remove you from the picture in order to focus on the other person. This can be difficult for some people, as they think that revealing their own experiences can help. While this may be true later, in the initial stages you really need to understand the problem, and

empathy:
understanding
another person's
point of view

this can only be done by listening carefully and providing encouraging verbal and non-verbal responses.

The following questions by Engleberg and Wynn (2015) provide a useful guide to understanding the range of empathic listening:

- Do you show interest in and concern about the other person?
- Does your non-verbal behaviour communicate friendliness and trust?
- Do you avoid highly critical reactions to others?
- Do you avoid talking about your own experiences and feelings when someone else is describing theirs?

Just attempting to understand will help to minimise the barriers, as the other person will usually appreciate the concern. Bramley and Matiti (2014) studied the impact of empathy and found that patients really appreciated nurses' empathetic behaviour; this not only related to their own care but also their observations of the care of other patients. They also wanted nurses who displayed little empathy to understand what it felt like to be nursed in an uncompassionate way. Empathy should not be confused with sympathy. Davies (2014) differentiates between them by analysing differences in terms of their impact. With sympathy, a patient will probably feel pitied, but if the patient is approached in an empathetic way, they are more likely to feel validated.

Validation

validation:
accepting what another person says as being valid to improve the flow of communication

Validation is linked to empathy, and it can be another useful strategy – particularly when dealing with patients and their families. Validation is accepting what people say or do 'as a valid expression of thought and feelings in that particular circumstance at that particular time' (Harvey & Ahmann, 2014, p. 143). This does not mean you have to agree with the other person, but simply that you acknowledge how they feel. For example, if you perceived a patient to be malingering, rather than dismissing the complaint you could accept that the patient may generally feel that way and acknowledge it to the patient. This can then help to negotiate the communication until a solution is found.

Empathy is largely considered to be a positive trait. Consider what problems might be associated with it.

Interpersonal barriers

Interpersonal barriers are the barriers that arise between people. If two or more people interact in a professional or personal capacity, it is unlikely that some kind of interpersonal barrier will occur. However, as we have all experienced, interpersonal barriers can and do happen. There are a number of particular variables that can contribute to interpersonal barriers in the nursing context. One of the biggest can arise from cultural, gender and hierarchical differences and misunderstandings.

interpersonal barriers: barriers between people, such as gender, status and culture

Culture

As discussed in Chapters 2 and 5, the ways in which people interact are largely driven by their cultural background. There can be subtle or obvious differences that can thwart effective communication for nursing students. Differences in social manners can create warped perceptions about others that can lead to a breakdown in communication. Nursing students need to be mindful of these differences so they can negotiate common understanding and help the other person to be more aware of how their actions may be perceived by others. For example, in some cultures saying 'please' and 'thank you' is an alien concept. This is because such niceties are implicit in the message and saying them would seem to be redundant (Okougha & Tilki, 2010). However, to the Australian nurse, not using these terms appears to reflect arrogance or even hostility. Chapter 5 discusses these cultural barriers in more depth.

Gender

Although people strive to be gender-neutral in the professional context, the reality is that the sex of the communicator can have a significant impact. Male and female nursing students will be faced with patients who would prefer not to have them as their nurse. This can be upsetting to the student, and can create interpersonal difficulties. The student may take offence and feel rejected by the patient, but often there are underlying cultural or personal reasons that go beyond merely being a difficult patient. Some patients have been traumatised by earlier events and this trauma can re-emerge when they are at their most vulnerable, both physically and psychologically. Teshuva and Wells (2014) found that Holocaust survivors had different triggers that could bring back distressing wartime experiences and create a reaction to being cared for by males:

> A Holocaust survivor explained that it was important for her to be assisted in the toilet by a female carer because during the war she and her fellow concentration camp inmates had suffered the daily humiliation of having to go to the toilet out in the open in full view of men. (Teshuva & Wells, 2014, p. 531)

This is an example where extreme trauma has created a challenging problem, and there is a clear need for a healthcare professional to deliver understanding, sensitivity and support to their patient. In a situation like this, the nurse must try to realise that the reaction is not about him personally, but rather about a broader psychological issue. There are numerous other fundamental issues that male nurses need to face in dealing with patients who are not traumatised:

> Gender stereotypes that distance men from physical nurturing have constructed a discourse in which it is acceptable for female nurses to intimately touch patients, but it is strange for men to do so. Since people have been conditioned from childhood to expect such behavior from women, such care from a man can lead to feelings of discomfort for both parties … (Harding, North & Perkins, 2008, p. 89)

This stereotyping and its consequent impact on interpersonal communication with patients could be inhibiting patient care – particularly intimate care. The number of male nurses has been surprisingly stable in Australia, with the proportion only changing from 9 per cent in 2001 to 10 per cent a decade later, in 2011. The gender imbalance for doctors, however, has been improving during that time period, and the numbers of women in the younger cohort of doctors have increased to 57 per cent (ABS, 2013). Unlike other professions, the numbers of male nurses are still not large, and this fact can make them appear to be still a 'novelty' – particularly in the hospital setting. Like women, men choose nursing to help others, and when this care is rejected there can be a negative emotional response. It is interesting to note there is not the same response to a male doctor's touch because his touch has been normalised (Harding, North & Perkins, 2008). This may explain why higher numbers of complaints are made about male nurses regarding minor boundary violations. What is considered an acceptable degree of involvement by a female nurse may be perceived as over-involved and unacceptable in a male nurse; this suggests that there is still some anxiety about men in nursing (Chiarella & Adrian, 2013). An understanding of this interpersonal barrier can alert the nurse to a possible cause of patient discomfort.

Hierarchy

Many large organisations need a tightly structured hierarchy to ensure tasks are clearly outlined and efficiently completed; however, problems can occur when there are significant status differences. For instance, hierarchical differences between health workers – particularly between senior physicians and nurses/nursing students – may result in a nurse's reluctance to contradict the physician. This is illustrated in the following real-life situation:

> A patient experiences the sudden onset of supraventricular tachycardia, and a multidisciplinary clinical team responds. During the course of treatment, the physician team leader mistakenly orders amiodarone intravenous push rather than adenosine. Although team members are concerned about the appropriateness of this order, they choose not to speak up. The drug is given, resulting in severe hypotension and bradycardia. This real case illustrates the difficulty of challenging an authority figure even when significant negative consequences could result, a phenomenon that has been observed in … myriad … differing domains. (Calhoun et al., 2013, p. 13)

Strategies to overcome interpersonal barriers

There are many strategies that can be used to minimise interpersonal barriers, although there are so many variables within any communication event that their success can be mixed. One of the most powerful strategies stems from *self-awareness* and *awareness*. Both are needed to measure just how effective communication is. Nursing students need to be mindful and watchful, and generally build an awareness of their own backgrounds and experiences, which can lead to the development of intrapersonal barriers.

Assertiveness

People have a range of communication styles ranging from passiveness to aggression. Both these styles have potential problems because they are not based on equitable foundations, but rather on a power imbalance. Assertiveness, which is somewhere in the middle of these two extremes, is a more effective style in most circumstances. This is because assertiveness is based on mutual respect – respect for you and respect for the other person involved. An assertive person is direct and honest, and can say 'no' without feeling guilty. With this style, you stand up for your rights but try to understand the other person's viewpoint. You also end the discussion with what you want done.

Case study

The following brief scenario explains how Angus gets his point across without undermining Jack:

Angus: Jack, I waited an hour for you to turn up for our appointment this morning. I had to reschedule several things to make sure I could be there. I was stuck in traffic on the way back and ended up wasting several hours. This is extremely frustrating given the deadlines that are looming. (*State the problem*)

Jack: Sorry Angus, I just forgot. I've been so busy. (*Listen*)

Angus: I know that you're busy but you've now created more problems for me. (*Empathise* but let the other person know that there has been an impact)

Jack: I can only apologise again, Angus.

Angus: Let's forget about it now, Jack. In the future, though, please make sure you turn up or you give me plenty of warning that the meeting has to be rescheduled. (*Propose a solution to avoid further incidents*)

Critical reflection

》》 Reflect on an interpersonal problem you are experiencing or have experienced. Explain how using the above scenario may have helped you to resolve the situation.

The most important part of all assertive behaviour is to take the emotion out of the situation. If there is a calmness underpinning the conversation, it can often lead to more meaningful solutions. Without self-control, the problem can snowball into something that will be much more difficult to resolve.

Despite this, assertiveness may not be the best communicating style in every situation. There may be a need for a passive approach to appease a patient who is potentially violent until the patient is in a calmer frame of mind. Conversely, aggression may be needed in some situations, although this would be rare. Such a situation could occur if a health and safety issue were involved, and you needed to act very quickly without time to explain. The style you use depends on the variables. The nurse needs to think about styles and be adaptable to the situation. The term 'assertiveness' can often be confused with 'aggressiveness', but with assertiveness the situation does not finish with one person being the victor, but rather focuses on ways to calmly expose the problem and find solutions.

Graded assertiveness

As mentioned above, nurses can often be intimidated by the hierarchical structure of their healthcare environment. Physicians and senior nurses may be intimidating to a new nurse who may not be able to challenge instructions, despite the possibility of risks for patients. Mistakes can be made because of the timidity of nurses, and therefore techniques need to be consciously explored to help with the situation. One technique that can help is graded assertiveness. This is an approach that starts with a gentle nudge to the supervisor or physician to alert them to a problem with the current treatment. This may be all that is required (Curtis, Tzannes & Rudge, 2011). If the point isn't accepted, the nurse can then go to the next step or grade to try to get their point across. This stepped process can take the stress out of the situation for the nurse, as not all the steps may be needed to be effective. Table 2.1 illustrates how graded assertiveness could work:

TABLE 2.1 *An example of graded assertiveness*

Level 1: express initial concern with an 'I' statement.	I am concerned about …
Level 2: make an inquiry or offer a solution.	Would you like me to …?
Level 3: ask for an explanation.	It would help me to understand …
Level 4: a definitive challenge demanding a response.	For the safety of patient you must listen to me.

Source: Curtis, Tzannes & Rudge (2011, p. 18) © International Council of Nurses

You can see that the steps start out in a relatively benign way, but progress to using more direct language. You will note, however, that the levels never spill over into aggressive behaviour, but rather remain assertive throughout.

Rebecca's story

Case study

I had only been nursing for a few months, and I became very friendly with one of the patients, a woman who had children around my age, and we soon developed a friendly rapport. She came to trust and respect me, and she eventually revealed something that could have had implications for her treatment. She said she was too scared to tell the doctor, who was particularly imposing and quite scary! I told her not to worry, and that I would talk to him. The problem was that I felt just as intimidated as the patient. I tried several times to tell him, but he dismissed me and walked away. I really felt that I'd let my patient down and I knew her well-being was my main responsibility. Unfortunately, she witnessed my ineffectual attempts and, although she smiled weakly at me, I knew she was disappointed. This somehow gave me the courage to seek out the doctor and, after some embarrassing attempts to articulate the problem, I finally managed to get my point across. He eventually listened and understood the problem, and immediately went back to talk to the patient. A potentially dangerous situation was averted, but I vowed that I would overcome my mousy behaviour and stand up for my patients, no matter how awkward I felt. The funny thing is that it became easier as time went on, and I became an effective advocate for my patients; it eventually became quite natural. I also noticed a distinct change in the medical staff's reaction to me. They actually sought out my advice!

Critical reflection

>> Reflect on a situation where you have used graded assertiveness. In the nursing context, this is called advocacy; it is one of the codes of practice.

Structured communication

The medical community is constantly striving to make its communication as efficient as possible. Handover between health professionals is one area that has been studied and improved through application of theory to practice, and the methods used have been refined to achieve optimum effectiveness. One of the more recent methods is ISBAR, which developed from SBAR. ISBAR is a mnemonic that stands for Introduction, Situation, Background, Assessment and Recommendation. The term 'ISBAR' is useful even at a superficial level, as most medical staff find it easy to remember (Finnigan, Marshall & Flanagan, 2010). It helps to provide consistent information that can help nurse-to-nurse, nurse-to-doctor and nurse-to-paramedic communication in the handover of patients, and help to improve the confidence of all involved. It is a template that helps nurses and paramedics focus their thinking and convey a clear message. Because it involves a protocol that can be learnt, it thus reduces **semantic barriers** (see below), and helps to prevent intrapersonal or interpersonal barriers. ISBAR helps to 'flatten' hierarchy, minimise assumptions and create common expectations (Dawson, King & Grantham, 2013). Below is an example of how ISBAR works:

semantic barriers: misunderstanding created by the use of words such as jargon or specialised language

Case study

A woman has begun vomiting blood in the hallway of her home. Her teenage daughter is at home and rings for an ambulance. When the ambulance arrives, paramedics find the woman cyanosed and, after checking the patient's vitals, have to administer oxygen and fluids. They transport the woman to the local hospital. The following is the ISBAR exchange between Accident & Emergency (A&E) doctors and nurses during handover in preparation for the end of a shift in A&E:

ACRONYM	STEPS	EXAMPLE
I	Introduction	I'm Dr James Williams. This is patient Patricia O'Reilly.
S	Situation	Patricia is a 54-year-old female who has presented with hematemesis and has been vomiting dark red blood and large clots approximately 10–15 centimetres in diameter. Paramedics brought her in about half an hour ago; they estimated by the amount of blood on the floor that she'd lost about 2000 millilitres of blood. When she arrived, the patient showed signs of hypovolemic shock including central cyanosis and tachycardia with marked tachypnea, so we administered oxygen and fluids and bloods via a central venous catheter in the neck. She was in a confused state and her skin was cool and pale. Her pulse is currently 130 bpm; blood pressure is 90/60. We've organised full bloods – CBC [complete blood count], clotting tests, liver function tests and blood chemistries.
B	Background	Her daughter reports she'd been feeling nauseous this morning and went to the toilet about an hour ago. After leaving the toilet, she stated that she felt ill and then collapsed to the floor while vomiting blood. Her daughter immediately called paramedics. Her daughter said she has never vomited blood before; she's had no nosebleeds or surgeries. She's not had any recent dental work and has no history of stomach problems. Her daughter said Patricia's only health problem has been a persistently very sore arm for the past few months which she has sought medical assistance about from her GP.
A	Assessment	This might be referred pain: we suspect a gastro-intestinal bleed, possibly from an ulcer or neoplasm since her abdomen is still palpable and soft.
R	Recommendation	We need to organise an emergency endoscopy with a possible laparotomy and further surgery.

More experienced health workers may follow these procedures automatically, but when there is a common technique employed, such as ISBAR, each person knows what is expected and this reduces the risk of mistakes.

Semantic barriers

The healthcare world is often complex and confronting for patients, and semantic barriers can add to this anxiety. Semantic barriers relate to misunderstanding of words. This can be due to the use of specialised language such as medical jargon or it could be connotation relating to language. Connotation relates to the emotional impact behind words: the same word can be perceived in very different ways by patients, depending on their field of experience. For example, if a doctor or nurse stated that a particular physical symptom could be indicative of an underlying mental disorder, the impact could vary. One patient could pursue the conversation in a curious way to explore the condition; another could immediately respond to the 'underlying mental disorder' term, which could be a trigger word leading to self-labelling and unnecessary distress.

Medical jargon is necessary. It is not designed to deliberately distance the medical staff from the patient; however, this can often be the unintended effect. It is shorthand to convey a great deal of knowledge into single words, although they are often not simple words. Some terms such as 'BP' for 'blood pressure' are easily understood, but when nurses and doctors use terms such as 'bibasilar' (lung function) or 'ganglioneuromas' (rare tumours) this creates obvious barriers to understanding the message being conveyed. Additionally, it can become even more confusing when acronyms such as 'DTR' (deep tendon reflexes) are used. Despite these problems, jargon and acronyms are necessary as they contain a wealth of complex meaning beneath them and this will of course move the diagnosis and treatment phases along much more quickly and efficiently. However, this does not discount the fear and anxiety such specialised language can create in the patient, for in that moment they are the outsider looking in and there can be a sense of alienation despite being the focus of the medical discussion. Nurses from other countries will have an added layer of semantic complexity. Like other nurses, they face the medical jargon and technical terms, but they also have to deal with more fundamental semantic challenges. (See Chapter 5 for a discussion of cross-cultural nursing.)

Use of words can also create problems in unexpected ways. Because nursing students or new nurses have a great deal of information with which to grapple, they may be conscious that they have to give the patient all the necessary information. However, an Australian study has shown that over-explaining some situations can reflect a lack of sensitivity to some patients. The researchers argue that it is important for nurses to be able to gauge patient readiness for information (O'Hagan et al., 2011). Handover procedures have changed over time, with many handovers now taking place in front of the patient, and this change has created both benefits and problems. The benefits are that the patient feels part of the process and may feel less vulnerable being a more active participant and being able to alert nurses to any misinformation that may have crept into the process. It also helps to reassure the patients that the nurses have enough information about their presentation, condition and plan, which in turn reassures them that the nurses will have enough detail to competently care for them; the patient also feels a sense of importance (Kerr et al., 2013). However, the situation can also create semantic barriers, as the patient will not be able to understand the specialised language needed for an effective and efficient handover. Lu, Kerr and McKinlay (2014) confirmed the problem with using medical jargon in a study where they analysed patient perceptions of the handover. One of the interesting findings was that some patients thought the medical jargon not only distanced them from the process, but they were concerned that inexperienced nurses did not understand the terms as well.

Strategies to overcome semantic barriers

Empathy (discussed above) seems to be an odd strategy for what appears to be a language issue. However, if doctors or nurses have an understanding of the impact of jargon or technical terms on the patient, they may temper their linguistic behaviour and try to adjust their approach by clearly explaining pathology and procedures.

Audience analysis

Audience analysis is used widely in marketing and public relations, and it may seem out of place when discussing barriers in the nursing world. Audience analysis is finding out about your audience (or receiver) to tailor a message in order to make it more effective. For communication specialists, audience analysis requires a deliberate and structured approach to gaining demographic and psychographic information about a group of people. For example, advertisers will find out demographic information (statistical information such as age, sex, occupation and race) and psychographic data (values and attitudes) to ascertain whether their products are a good 'match' to the facts found in their audience analysis. This necessarily becomes an exercise based on generalisations, and even stereotyping, because the advertisers cannot tweak every communication to a particular person, although they are trying to do so through the use of social media.

The basic idea of audience analysis is important to nurses and nursing students, although they will not use such a structured approach as professional communicators. However, they can find out as much information as possible to try to understand their colleagues and patients so they can respond in a way that will be useful. The nurse will already have access to demographic information, but it is the psychographic information that can often drive communication. For example, as mentioned elsewhere in this chapter, some knowledge about a person's experience can help the nurse to understand the patient's attitude to nursing care. Also, if a nurse has intrapersonal barriers such as stereotyping, bias or prejudice, gaining such knowledge can help to develop empathy by gaining insights into other people's lives.

Physical/external barriers

Physical barriers are anything in the environment that negatively affects the communication process. This may include inadequate or too much time, a lack of resources, the physical environment, physical disability and a negative appearance (for example, a rude gesture or angry face). Nursing students will be well aware of a constant physical barrier in their student lives – lack of time. With one of the busiest study programs to contend with, they may unwittingly be preparing themselves for the reality of busy hospitals which are often subject to heavy workloads, and this can compromise the quality of the time spent on their duties, particularly with patients.

> **physical barriers:** any environmental or resource issues that affect the physical comfort or health of people, ultimately weakening the communication process

The use of time is a form of non-verbal communication (chronemics), and how people use it can be telling. Hemsley, Balandin and Worrall (2012) explored time as a resource in a very interesting way in a study of nursing patients with complex communication needs: specifically, patients with developmental disorders or little to no functional speech. The study found nurses were adept at prioritising and managing time, but a lack of time in these circumstances often reflected negative attitudes and emotions to the problem. They also found nurses had many external barriers that could compromise their job, such as the ever-increasing funding pressures on the Australian health system, where budget cutting is seen as more important than health funding.

The problem with time pressure is that it can affect patient care. Nurses need to remain task orientated because of competing time pressures, and patient care can sometimes be delivered in an impersonal manner because of these pressures (Chan, Jones & Wong, 2013). Time pressure can also lead to mundane consequences, such as not having time to eat lunch; however, the long-term consequence could be physical and psychological problems, particularly regarding stress (Applebaum et al., 2010). Time is a physical barrier that can lead to intrapersonal barriers, which can ultimately affect professional competence. Nurses' perceived lack of confidence and time to discuss emotional issues with patients, as well as broader concerns regarding the stigma surrounding depression, also present potential obstacles to effective recognition of depression in these settings. Furthermore, the difficulty in differentiating clinical depression from grief reactions represents another potential barrier to the recognition of depressive symptoms, and ultimately the provision of pathways to care (McCabe et al., 2012). This further demonstrates how intertwined the barriers can be.

Other physical barriers include issues relating to resources. These can include low nurse-to-patient ratios, shiftwork issues, leave and pay. A poor skill-mix also adds to nurses' stress as handovers are more time-consuming. Nursing students are also sometimes used as 'staff', which is inappropriate in the Australian context (Dawson et al., 2014). Despite increases in some groups' staff in Dawson and colleagues' study, the nurse-to-patient ratio often remained low because of absenteeism. Staff shortages can therefore lead to lower levels of job satisfaction and increased workloads. Ultimately, this can affect patient care (Dawson et al., 2014).

Casual staffing

Budget cuts often mean an increase in casual staffing. According to Batch, Barnard and Windsor (2009), this creates problems such as nursing staff not having enough familiarity with what is happening because of a lack of continuity. This can have a direct negative impact on the quality of patient care. Nurses are working in unfamiliar situations, and have less opportunity to build rapport with patients (Batch, Barnard & Windsor, 2009). Part-time staffing can also compromise quality of information – for example, part-time nurses are 'less likely to be included in team handovers which might limit their opportunity for education and compromise the quality of information transfer at handover' (Street et al., 2011, p. 138).

The physical environment can also create problems. If architects or management are aware of potential problems, they can incorporate changes into future design modifications to avoid pitfalls. For example, Teshuva and Wells (2014) found that some design features of the built environment in long-term care facilities can potentially trigger traumatic memories for some patients, such as those who are survivors of war. Enclosed spaces, long corridors and locked windows and doors can elicit memories of oppression.

Strategies to overcome physical barriers

The strategies needed to address physical barriers are often beyond the scope of the nursing staff, as resource issues such as staffing and scheduling are the responsibility of management. However, if there is an environmental factor that is clearly affecting the comfort of patients and/or colleagues, the most obvious strategy is to provide or seek feedback. Chapter 3 discusses feedback in some depth. If there are no positive results from the feedback, then assertiveness, graded assertiveness and even elements of ISBAR could be applied.

Case study

Peter had worked in the hospital wards for six months. He had done extremely well in his nursing studies, and had high expectations for his new career. He was enthusiastic and committed to learning as much as he could. This was short-lived, however, as almost from the start he perceived negative attitudes from his supervisors, from some of the doctors and even from his patients. He was given the worst shifts, and he seemed to be overloaded with tasks that he couldn't possibly achieve. He later learnt that his supervisor had been bad-mouthing him, making fun of his high achievements and calling him 'Wonder Boy' in a sarcastic tone. The supervisor's attitude was conveyed to the doctors, who also treated him with less respect than he deserved. In addition, he was rejected by both female and male patients who wanted female nurses. He became depressed and was starting to think his training had been a waste of time and money.

Critical reflection

》》 In the above scenario, identify the symptoms of the problem and link each symptom to a broader communication barrier. How would you try to minimise each barrier?

Summary

This chapter has explored the idea of theory being a stepping-stone to developing practical problem-solving tools in the nursing context. Communication theory was introduced, together with a theoretical explanation of what happens when we communicate by way of the three models of communication: the linear, interactive and transactional models. Each of these models added to the explanation of communication theory, demonstrating that theory can evolve and be improved with each iteration. The transactional model, which is essentially based on perception, is the most appropriate way of explaining communication and the elements of barriers (noise), field of experience and context, and can be used as a prism to explore the multifaceted nursing communication processes. Once communication barriers – intrapersonal, interpersonal, semantic or physical – are analysed, different strategies – empathy, audience analysis and structured communication such as ISBAR – can be applied. Therefore, while theory may be dismissed as being irrelevant or an academic indulgence, it helps us to explore our world, and can have a profound effect on the nursing community, as it is the prerequisite for problem-solving in hospital wards and other healthcare settings.

Discussion and critical thinking questions

2.1 Think about an interpersonal clash you've had in your personal or professional lives. Do you think that this was a result of intrapersonal barriers of one or both parties? How would you try to resolve this kind of problem in the future?

2.2 Have you noticed a consistent pattern of behaviour by patients, colleagues or fellow students in relation to how they respond to an event? Try to develop a broad theory as a way of explaining this behaviour.

2.3 In your lectures, are you overwhelmed by the amount of jargon or unfamiliar words? What is a way you can overcome this linguistic hurdle?

2.4 As an advocate for patient care, you will need to learn to be assertive. As an initial exercise, apply the graded assertiveness approach to a problem you face. Start with a problem that is not critical. Once you've done this, evaluate the situation from your perspective and in terms of solving the problem.

Learning extension

Think of a clinical environment in which you have worked. Is the communication in this environment always effective? Have you ever thought, 'Why are they communicating in this way?' Have you considered how people could improve their communication? Choose one of the situations that could be improved (for example, handovers). What could you do to improve the communication? If you had the chance to go back to this clinical area, what ideas might you have for communicating differently?

Further reading

Levett-Jones, T. (2013). *Critical conversations for patient safety: An essential guide for health professionals.* Sydney: Pearson Education. This Australian text addresses the communication between health professionals and the critical relationship between communication and patient safety.

References

Al Abed, N.A., Hickman, L., Jackson, D., DiGiacomo, M. & Davison, P.M. (2014). Older Arab migrants in Australia: Between the hammer of prejudice and the anvil of social isolation. *Contemporary Nurse*, 46(20): 259–62.

Applebaum, D., Fowler, S., Fiedler, N., Omowunmi, O. & Robson, M. (2010). The impact of environmental factors on nursing stress, job satisfaction, and turnover intention. *The Journal of Nursing Administration*, 40(7/8): 323–8.

Australian Bureau of Statistics (ABS) (2013). *Australian social trends*. Cat no. 4102.0. Canberra: ABS.

Batch, M., Barnard, A. & Windsor, C. (2009). Who's talking? Communication and the casual/part-time nurse: A literature review. *Contemporary Nurse*, 33(1): 20–9.

Birks, M., Missen, K., Al-Motlaq, M. & Marino, E. (2014). Babies and machines that go 'beep': First-year nursing students' preferred areas of future practice. *International Journal of Nursing Practice*, 20: 353–9.

Bramley, L. & Matiti, M. (2014). How does it really feel to be in my shoes? Patients' experiences of compassion within nursing care and their perceptions of developing compassionate nurses. *Journal of Clinical Nursing*, 23: 2790–9.

Calhoun, A.W., Boone, M., Miller, K. & Pian-Smith, M.C. (2013). Case and commentary: Using simulation to address hierarchy issues during medical crises. *The Journal of the Society for Simulation in Healthcare*, 8(1): 13–19.

Chan, E.A., Jones, A. & Wong, K. (2013), The relationships between communication, care and time are intertwined: A narrative inquiry exploring the impact of time on registered nurses' work. *Journal of Advanced Nursing*, 69(9): 2020–9.

Chiarella, M. & Adrian, A. (2013). Boundary violations, gender and the nature of nursing work. *Nursing Ethics*, 21(3): 267–77.

Curtis, K., Tzannes, A. & Rudge, T. (2011). How to talk to doctors: A guide for effective communication. *International Nursing Review*, 58: 13–20.

Davies, N. (2014). Empathic nursing: Going the extra mile. *Practice Nursing*, 25(4): 198–202.

Dawson, A.J., Stasa, H., Roche, M.A., Homer, C.S. & Duffield, C. (2014). Nursing churn and turnover in Australian hospitals: Nurses' perceptions and suggestions for supportive strategies. *BMC Nursing*, 13: 11.

Dawson, S., King, L. & Grantham, H. (2013). Review article: Improving the hospital clinical handover between paramedics and emergency department staff in the deteriorating patient. *Emergency Medicine Australasia*, 25: 393–405.

Engleberg, I.N. & Wynn, D.R. (2015). *Think communication*. Boston: Pearson Education.

Finnigan, M.A., Marshall, S.D. & Flanagan, B.T. (2010). ISBAR for clear communication: One hospital's experience spreading the message. *Australian Health Review*, 34: 400–4.

Griffin, E. (2009). *Communication communication communication: A first look at communication theory*, 7th edn. Boston: McGraw-Hill.

Harding, T., North, N. & Perkins, R. (2008). Sexualizing men's touch: Male nurses and the use of intimate touch in clinical practice. *Research and Theory for Nursing Practice*, 22(2): 88–102.

Harvey, P. & Ahmann, E. (2014). Validation: A family-centred communication skill. *Family Matters*, 40(3): 143–7.

Hemsley, B., Balandin, S. & Worrall, I. (2012). Nursing the patient with complex communication needs: Time as a barrier and a facilitator to successful communication in hospital. *Journal of Advanced Nursing*, 68(1): 116–26.

Jirwe, M., Gerrish, K. & Emami, A. (2010). Student nurses' experiences of communication in cross-cultural care encounters. *Scandinavian Journal of Caring Sciences*, 24: 436–44.

Kerr, D., McKay, K., Klim, S., Kelly, A. & McCann, T. (2013). Attitudes of emergency department patients about handover at the bedside. *Journal of Clinical Nursing*, 23: 1685–93.

Lu, S., Kerr, D. & McKinlay, L. (2014). Bedside nursing handover: Patients' opinions. *International Journal of Nursing Practice*, 20: 451–9.

McCabe, M.P., Mellor, T.E., Hallford, D.J. & Goldhammer, D.L. (2012). Detecting and managing depressed patients: Palliative care nurses' self-efficacy and perceived barriers to care. *Journal of Palliative Medicine*, 15(4): 463–7.

O'Hagan, S., Manias, E., Elder, C., Pill, J., Woodward-Kron, R., McNamara, T., Webb, G. & McColl, G. (2011). What counts as effective communication in nursing? Evidence from nurse educators' and clinicians' feedback on nurse interactions with simulated patients. *Journal of Advanced Nursing*, 70(6): 1344–56.

Okougha, M. & Tilki, M. (2010). Experience of overseas nurses: The potential for misunderstanding. *British Journal of Nursing*, 19(2): 102–6.

Price, B. (2013). Countering the stereotype of the unpopular patient. *Nursing Older People*, 25(6): 27–34.

Shannon, C.E. & Weaver, W. (1949). *A mathematical model of communication*. Urbana, IL: University of Illinois Press.

Spiteri, D. (2013). Can my perceptions of the 'other' change? Challenging prejudices against migrants amongst adolescent boys in a school for low achievers in Malta. *Research in Education*, 89: 41–60.

Street, M., Eustace, P., Livingston, P.M., Craike, M.J., Kent, B. & Patterson, D. (2011). Communication at the bedside to enhance patient care: A survey of nurses' experience and perspective of handover. *International Journal of Nursing Practice*, 17: 133–40.

Teshuva, K. & Wells, Y. (2014). Experiences of ageing and aged care in Australia of older survivors of genocides. *Ageing and Society*, 34(3): 518–37.

Wittenberg-Lyles, E., Goldsmith, J. & Ferrell, B. (2013). Oncology nurse communication barriers to patient-centered care. *Clinical Journal of Oncology Nursing*, 17(2): 152–8.

Wood, J. (2013). *Interpersonal communication: Everyday encounters*. Independence, KY: Cengage.

Building lifelong learning capacities and resilience in changing academic and healthcare contexts

3

Jill Lawrence

Learning objectives

- Appreciate your awareness of self and understand its impact on your assumptions, expectations and beliefs.

- Identify the languages and behaviours of the new academic context you are entering.

- Identify the practices and strategies that can enhance your transition to the new academic context.

- Apply two models of transition to your studies as you progress through your university degree.

- Identify the efficacy of the models in terms of your capabilities for lifelong learning and resilience.

Key terms

- Context
- Cultural practices
- Culture
- Jargon
- Literacies
- Power relationships

Introduction

Chapter 1 introduced you to the impact of your awareness of self and the factors that motivated you to undertake study and work in nursing and healthcare. Chapter 2 then presented the concepts of perception and world-view, and examined how these influence your communication using the theoretical perspective provided by communication theory. The chapter also investigated how the expectations, assumptions, stereotypes and prejudices we have inside us can lead to intrapersonal communication barriers and prevent us from communicating effectively. Chapter 5 will explore these concepts further by discussing cross-cultural awareness, which asks you to think about your sense of self in relation to your cultural understandings and beliefs. Chapter 6 then describes how nurses' self-concept and self-efficacy can influence the effectiveness of their communication, which in turn influences the effectiveness of their clinical care.

Awareness of self is so important that it is a central concept in other theoretical perspectives. For example, in psychological theory, awareness of self is described as self-concept, identity or self-efficacy. In sociological theory, it is identified as your 'way of knowing' or discourses. Thus the same concept has different connotations and applications in different theoretical perspectives.

This chapter expands on Chapters 1 and 2 by exploring further how our awareness of self influences our capacity to adapt, or make a comfortable transition, to the new university culture. It does this by helping you to further explore your own self-awareness and assisting you to identify the practices, literacies and languages that you will need to demonstrate if you are to be successful in the new higher education or university context. The twin concepts of awareness of self and awareness of context then form the foundation for two models of transition that are introduced at the end of the chapter. The case studies included in the chapter are the reflections of students studying a first-year, first-semester subject. The reflections were collected as part of a research study investigating the experiences of students as they began their studies at university.

Understanding who you are and what you bring to higher education

As you enter higher education, it is critical that you think about the experiences, skills, knowledge and understandings you bring with you. For example, as a result of your experiences and backgrounds, some of you are more familiar with higher education and its ways of doing things, while others are more unfamiliar or perhaps even challenged by the new higher education **culture**. Who

culture: what
people do every
day: how they
behave, speak,
relate and make
things

you are is, in fact, one of the biggest research areas in learning and teaching at higher education. Thirty years ago (up until the 1980s), the majority of higher education students were male, from higher socio-economic backgrounds, white and able-bodied (Schuetze & Slowey, 2000). Today, the cohort of students is far more diverse. Some are older and have been in the workforce for a number of years. Many come from different countries and cultures. Some may be the first in their family to attend higher education. Many are simultaneously working (perhaps in a full-time job) and/or balancing work, family and study. Some might have a number of children. Today's students are also studying in variety of ways – online, on campus or externally, or in all three modes simultaneously.

Case study

These are the reflections of six different students studying nursing who are completing the first weeks of their first semester of study at university.

- I'm 39 years old and mother of a 4-year-old boy and a girl of 15. I live outside a middle-sized country town. I am currently working at the base hospital as an AIN [Assistant in Nursing], and have always wanted to be a nurse. I am hoping to get my head around all this and do the best I can. When I get free time I love to spend time with my family, exploring different places, bush walking, and fishing, anything out doors.

- I am a second semester nursing student on campus. I come from China and I have been in Australia for four years. I live without my family here. I was a nurse in China before, but I want to be a registered nurse and get my nursing degree in Australia. I like to help people and communicate with them, when I see their smiling face I think this is the best reward I got. I have learned English for four years. I think the language is

my weakness for my study, but I study hard. I do not really have leisure time for myself because I work part time in a nursing home facility. Apart from that, I like reading, cooking, gardening and I go to a church regularly on Sunday if I do not work in the weekend. I am also a volunteer at my church if they need help. I meet my church friends in the church. That is a joyful time for me.

- I am 26 years old and I live 150 kilometres away with my dad and step mum. I am currently travelling 150 kilometres to attend uni but am looking into accommodation as the travel is starting to take its toll on me and it is only Week 1!! I am in my first semester and so far I am enjoying it but at the same time a bit overwhelmed. After I graduated high school in 2007 I moved to a small mining town. After years of hard work I was finally employed as a Health, Safety and Rehabilitation Coordinator at the underground coal mine. This role was extremely challenging but always very rewarding. The skills and knowledge I obtained while in this position will assist me in the future. After six long years away from home I have returned to study my true passion of nursing.

- I'm a 45-year-old mum of eight and have chosen nursing because my husband has MS and I care for him and would like to be able to do more for him. I enjoy reading so hopefully that will help me in my studies although it's been a long time since school for me. Nursing has always been something that I wanted to do. I am a very caring person and enjoy helping people. It is a very rewarding feeling. I hope to one day become a midwife/ paediatric nurse as I love working with children. This journey will be exciting as it will be nice to want to and enjoy going to work which I have not experienced in my previous positions. I find it hard to identify my strengths so I will share some of my weaknesses. Probably one of my biggest weaknesses is staying focused. Sometimes when I am reading, something will trigger me to think about something else and I will go in a different direction. Another weakness is getting motivated and organised. I lead a very busy life and the travel to and from uni does not help with motivation as I get very tired. This is something that I am going to work really hard on because I do want to get the best out of this course and I do want to achieve great things.

- I graduated as an EN in 2012. I am married, and have four children and some pets. I work part time with my husband in our own business, doing everything from spray-painting to advising on Work Health & Safety and ensuring all first aid protocols are met. For the past eight years I have been a volunteer with St John's Ambulance Event Health Services, where I mentor and train members and attend events such as V8 supercars, rodeos and school fetes, to provide first aid to event stakeholders and the general public. This work is what led me, with encouragement from my mentors, to enter into nursing, something I have wanted to do since I was a young child. I have decided to further my education because I want to expand my knowledge base and skill levels, and gain another level of understanding, and I love the learning environment. I have a love of our elders and the wisdom they impart.

- I have recently completed my studies to be an enrolled nurse. My aim is to give myself every opportunity to find an area of the health industry that really interests me. I'm not sure what that is exactly yet but completing the Bachelor of Nursing will reduce the barriers to finding whatever it is. One of my strengths is an excellent work ethic. I believe this will assist me with completing my studies to the best of my ability. The most important strategy for this semester will be organisation. I have a lot going on so I need to be extra diligent with organising my time so I am always on top of my studies and not writing forums after the due date.

Critical reflection

>> Identify the previous learning experiences revealed through these reflections.

>> Specify the challenges experienced by the students that could affect their studies.

>> Write down a reflection about who you are, your strengths and weaknesses, and the experiences that have contributed to your view of the world as you enter the higher education context.

While developing an understanding of *who you are* is very important to how successfully you can make a comfortable transition to successful study, understanding the requirements and expectations of the *higher education environment* or context you are entering is also critical. The next section will help you to understand some of the expectations the university has about how you will need to behave and perform in this context in order to achieve your goals and objectives.

Understanding the new higher education context

literacies: characteristics, understandings, expectations and ways of behaving or acting in a certain context or culture – for example, academic literacy and numeracy refer to the skills of being able to read, write and do maths

The higher education context can be visualised as being like a new culture (Chapter 5 will also develop this concept). Like any new culture, it has a number of characteristics and a range of understandings and expectations about how you need to act, behave and communicate if you are to be successful in your study. These ways of behaving or acting are also called various names. In education theory they are called **literacies** – for example, academic literacy and numeracy refer to the skills of being able to read, write and do maths. In sociological or cross-cultural theory, they are called **cultural practices** – for example, there are cultural practices related to marriage, giving birth and funerals. They can also be identified as languages – for example, administrative language.

cultural practices: the non-verbal and verbal behaviours and rituals that are shared by cultural groups or sub-groups

Case study

When I began this semester, I found it hard – especially with electronic communication. I honestly had issues finding my way in the study desk, the power points and the learning system as a whole. It actually took me some time to familiarise myself with the online forums throughout this semester.

One of the barriers I have had to overcome, other than lack of confidence in myself, was terminology. I found that the concepts being taught were the same as things I already knew, but they were just called something different.

Critical reflection

›› What have you noticed about the new higher education environment? Are there any barriers that you find surprising?

›› Are there any rules and regulations about how to behave?

›› Where do you find information about how to become familiar with these rules and regulations or overcome any barriers?

The university, or higher education institution, is a culture that actually comprises a range of subcultures. Each subject, discipline area, program, course or degree has its own practices, with its own particular language, or **jargon**. Each area of the university has its own ways of doing things, or cultural behaviours or practices. For example, there is the library with its practices – which are often called information or database literacies. There is academic integrity and its referencing practices; for instance the APA or Harvard systems of referencing.

> **jargon:** refers to the meanings of words and technical or specialised language shared by a specific cultural group or sub-group

There are the computer and learning management systems which have very technical specifications. Each university sporting or support club also has its own cultural practices. There is academic literacy, or how to write persuasive academic arguments that achieve high marks. Not to mention the administrative jargon or language: GPAs, course specifications, exemptions, academic misconduct procedures, etc. The case study above also refers to a range of other practices or behaviours that students need to understand and become confident in if they are to succeed at their studies. These include a range of organisational, social and personal practices – for example, time and stress management and achieving a work/life balance, which are often critical to your perseverance in study.

Case study

To enable to start developing their understanding of the new academic culture, first-year nursing students were asked to interview a more experienced student. Here are some of their findings:

- My interview subject was very interesting, and the one thing that stood out for me, that I didn't expect, was that good study habits don't always come automatically; it is something that comes with trial and error and is an individual process. My main strategy for this semester will be to organise my study area into subject groups rather than whole-semester groups, which was my previous practice, as this should make it easier to locate any research, notes, etc. that I may need for assignments or study. As I am someone that is a fan of the written word (the ones I physically write) and has never used Facebook and Twitter, etc. … and until this week had never posted anything anywhere except a big red mailbox. This course is helping me become familiar and hopefully competent at these new tasks, which will eventually enable me to manage my time more effectively. I hope I will be able to manage my time, interact with others on a professional level, work autonomously and for myself personally upgrade my meagre computing skills which are all essential skills that are needed to be a successful, competent nurse.

- I interviewed a graduate nurse who studied full time on campus while juggling two children and part-time employment. Most of her practical experience was in large hospitals, and since graduation she has been based in a rural community.

The most surprising thing I learnt from the interview was hearing how nurses in the varying hospital settings treated her differently as a work colleague and the role variation in each location. I intend to plan ahead as much as possible. Like the graduate nurse, I have children and part-time employment to consider so it is essential I organise my time effectively. I have written all assignment due dates in my diary and regularly check in with study desk for updates and notifications. I have not written academically for many years and I lack confidence with referencing so I look forward to improving these skills.

- I interviewed a second-year student who is studying a Bachelor of Nursing; her husband is also a nursing student. One surprising thing that I found was she and her husband felt exactly the same way as I'm feeling in my first year of nursing. They both stated that with time the nerves will subside and the excitement of learning new things and paving the way to our new-found career. Helen's strategies for keeping on track for studies are lots of coffee, a study buddy to help focus, ensure that tasks are in on time and not leaving things to the last minute.

- I interviewed a qualified registered nurse who graduated last year. It was really good to talk to someone who had already been through the whole process and survived!! It was interesting and also refreshing to know that she went through the same emotions that I am going through when she first started uni. So we are not alone and she assured me that it does get better. The best tip that she gave me was to stay organised. This is an area which I need to improve and think that if I can get organised it will assist in making my uni experience a lot better. Strategies that I am going to put in place is assigning myself studying time in my diary and trying to stick to it. Put a big calendar on my wall which outlines assignment due dates. I need to stay motivated and stay confident.

- I interviewed my husband who is a second-year student. One of the surprising things I learnt from the interview is the difference in our study styles. I am quite used to jumping around with three or four tasks at once whereas he really requires a good few hours in one sitting concentrating on the one subject. This semester I am actually going to try and take something from that and seek out a set time for me to do the work I need to do so it isn't being forgotten. I also intend to follow some advice he gave me last semester, which is to really look at previous assessments when studying for final exams. It helped last semester and will surely help this one too.

Critical reflection

>> Describe the issues that the student nurses find surprising about their interviewee's experiences of study.

>> List the strategies the students put in place to help them study more effectively as a result of their reflections.

Conceptualising transition

So far, we have discussed the role of the new student accessing the university or higher education context or culture, and bringing with them their own expectations, backgrounds and ways of behaving, and previous educational experiences. In order to succeed at their studies, the new student needs to understand, or become familiar with, the practices and behaviours in the higher education culture. They also need to master and demonstrate these practices. For example, in your first assessment – usually in Week 4 or 5 – you will need to be able to use the university computer systems, assignment submission software, referencing and academic writing skills.

As shown in Figure 3.1, the literacies or languages required are many and varied. Many are quite complex – for example, what is critical thinking and how do you do it? You will develop your understandings of some of the literacies throughout your whole degree and into your career: they take time to develop. Nevertheless, you need to understand that these literacies or practices exist, and that they may be unfamiliar and unexpected. It is also important to

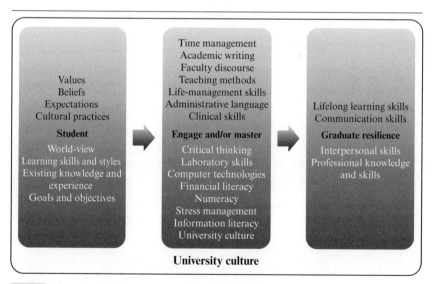

FIGURE 3.1 *Model for student transition*

understand that sources of help or information are readily available in the institution to support you. However, in order to take advantage of these resources, you do need to develop some practices or strategies of your own to use to access this support.

So what are the practices or strategies that will help you to become familiar with, engage in and master these cultural practices and behaviours? Again, they can be illustrated in a model (see Figure 3.2). This model presents three practical strategies that can assist you to make an effective transition to any new context or culture. These are reflective, communication and critical practices.

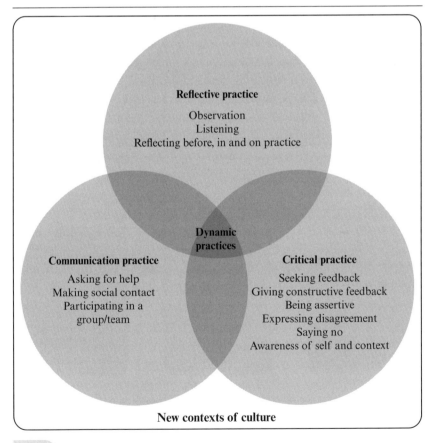

New contexts of culture

FIGURE 3.2   *Model for success strategies*
Source: Adapted from Lawrence (2009).

Reflective practice

The first practical strategy you can use to help you become comfortable with the new culture or context is your ability to reflect on the behaviours, languages or jargon of the context or culture. In a practical sense, this means that you need to observe, monitor, watch, listen to and reflect on others' behaviours and practices, and learn from your observations. In assessment terms, for example, how do you set out, structure, reference and write assignments? How do you submit them? Do you need a cover sheet and do you need to sign a statement that the assignment is your own work? Why do you need to do this? What happens if you don't? Where do you need to go to find out about these requirements? Is there an online source of help and assistance?

How do you write at university? Kossen, Kiernan and Lawrence (2013) suggest that one way to understand this is to watch how your lecturers and tutors write for you, and to analyse how the textbooks and research articles are written and set out, the kinds of information that are valued and whether, for example, they are peer reviewed (and what this means). Such observations provide a template of how your readers (your markers) want you to write for them. Samples or models help you to understand the kinds of formats to use, how to structure your writing, how to include graphs and figures, how to integrate tables and so on. Good observation techniques can save you a lot of time as well as help you to identify the group and/or individuals with whom you need to communicate in the new context (Kossen, Kiernan, Lawrence, 2013).

It is also important to recognise that if you do not know the practices in the new context you are not deficient, you are just unfamiliar. Korporaal (2014) provides the example of Ben Roberts-Smith, who spent 18 years in the military, served in Afghanistan six times, was a member of the elite Special Air Service (SAS), risked his life often and has been awarded a string of honours, including a Medal for Gallantry and a Victoria Cross. However, when he decided to do a higher education degree he had to learn to write essays and assignments:

> I don't have a degree. I have 18 years of experience in the military. I have written reports, I have done courses, I have studied everything from demolition to qualifications for being a paramedic, but I have never been involved with business. For me to come in here and do a 2500-word assignment, it's not something that I find is difficult to do, it's just that I have never done it before. Most people have been through this process before whereas for me it's a whole new learning process.

Case study

The nursing students now reflect on the university culture and the literacies and languages they need to exhibit if they are to succeed in their studies.

- This semester I have learnt many skills and strategies in a short amount of time. At the beginning of the semester I was unsure I would be able to take in so much information and remember it all but due to the learning strategies put in place by the lecturers and tutors I have managed to do just that. Many of my learning strengths have been expanded throughout the semester. For example, although I had knowledge of computer programs such as Microsoft Word before I started university, my knowledge of this and many other programs has increased and I have learnt handy techniques that I hadn't known about. This will help me considerably in the following subjects for this course.

- While I have a lot of learning strengths I still have some weaknesses that I need to work on. Time management is a weakness that I vowed I would have control of at the beginning of the semester; however, I still struggle with this. This weakness has caused me to have some late nights and I plan on not making this mistake again next semester. I feel my academic writing has greatly improved, although I still struggle with many aspects of essay writing and hope to improve on this more along with referencing. At the beginning of the semester referencing seemed daunting but now I somewhat enjoy it the more I understand how to do it correctly, but as I stated previously I have a lot of room for improvement.

- The results of the learning skills survey were very interesting and I think pretty close to the mark. I think it always helps to stand back and look at who you are and how you operate. Reflection like this often assists with making and accomplishing goals.

- In the beginning of this semester I was not so confident on online study as it was my first time studying an online course. I was worried about if something goes wrong how can I solve it, whom to ask and so many questions came around my mind. I am now more confident with online study as I learnt many things during this semester which helped me a lot. I found online tutors are really good who helped to clear my queries and it is easy to get access to them through email and forum. My aunt explained me about the advantages of online learning which encouraged me to study. Online learning saves time, cost and can study anywhere where there is internet access. It also helps to build self-confidence and encourages me to take responsibility for my learning.

Critical reflection

》》 Describe the techniques these students used to help them to reflect on their progress in their study.

》》 Name two of the challenges you faced at the beginning of the semester.

》》 Explain how these relate to the new or unexpected practices or requirements you needed to master in the university culture.

》》 Make a list of new practices and/or behaviours you have added to your repertoire in the weeks since you have started university.

Communication practice

The second practical tool relates to communication. As discussed throughout this book, you can choose to communicate in a range of different ways: via social network sites such as Instagram, Twitter and Facebook, and other media including portfolios, reports, oral presentations, teleconferencing, fax and email, media releases and so on. Communicating effectively will help you to gain and develop an understanding of the new culture being engaged with as well as the specific behaviours and practices of the culture (Kossen, Kiernan & Lawrence, 2013). The specific communication strategies that we discuss here are seeking help and information, participating in a group or team, and making social contact and conversation (Kossen, Kiernan & Lawrence, 2013).

Seeking help and information

Seeking help and information is an important communication strategy, which cannot be underestimated. The evidence from daily life is overwhelming. Kids Help Lines assist younger people to cope with changes in their lives. Cancer Support groups are set up to help people diagnosed with cancer to develop sources of support and information. Most higher education institutions have many sources of help available on campus and, increasingly, online.

Case study

- When I first started university this semester, I felt very anxious regarding obtaining digital literacy skills to aid in achieving optimal outcomes with my studies. My first engagement as an external student was to obtain skills in utilising the university's website. I achieved this by requesting a past USQ student to guide me through the basics. I found this strategy extremely helpful to get me started on the right track. To this day I am still learning new areas of the website that I was not originally aware of. I continue to learn this by exploring the website. The engagement of online forums and posts have also assisted in problem areas I have come across regarding digital literacy, and is great for student support.

- I would admit it has been difficult to understand some of the strong ethnic accents when some students talk. I don't want to appear rude but I have to ask them to repeat what they have said. One of our Indian CNs [clinical nurses] wasn't able to communicate with an old digger who was being quite rude and abusive to her. She asked me if I would assist him as there was not going to be the opportunity for her to do so as he was not going to change his mind. She wasn't upset or angry, she tried, she handed over and all was good, because I was able to culturally communicate with him, as I am Australian, from the bush with a military background. Nurses need to work with the understanding that no two persons are the same and communication and respect are important.

- I find it really helps to actively communicate with my student peers and find that everyone is happy to share experiences and help where they can, especially if you've missed something or don't understand. The meet-ups (student support peers) are also a fantastic way to gain knowledge from higher year students. I think the online forums are a great way to communicate with peers and teachers, especially if you need a question answered.

- I found that, working for Blue Care and in the hospital, the problem with communication is either with the patient or client (most elderly) who is hard to understand as they are unable to speak clearly and unable to voice their concerns. Or that information was not handed over properly, as staff are usually flat out and under-staffed. I find it's better to go to the patient's care plan or file and look at progress notes, thus getting a basic detail of the history of the person. I feel if we just take a little bit of time and to listen to others we might hear something others can't hear.

- When it came to learning how to use my actual computer effectively, my eldest daughter has taught me what I have needed to know such as how to find files and other items stored on my computer, how to create documents, how to fix problems that might occur on my computer such as internet connection problem. She showed me how to put my photo on the computer for my e-portfolio and how to attach files properly. Other sources of help have been classmates and using Google. It's very handy having young people in the house these days, as most are tech savvy. When Grandma needs help with the iPhone or Facebook, ask your 11-year-old to help her!

Critical reflection

>> Explore your higher education institution's website to locate sources of help for developing some of these practices. For example, does the library offer any classes or online tutorials? Is there help available about your learning management system – either technical assistance or learning management assistance?

It is important to reflect on your own attitude to asking for help. Some people don't find it easy to ask for help. Kossen, Kiernan and Lawrence (2013) suggest that some people may believe asking for help is a sign of weakness, while others may feel that they lack the confidence to ask. Some might be reluctant to ask because they are overconfident about their own abilities, while others may feel they do not have the 'right', or believe that they could be considered 'stupid', or they may equate help as 'remedial'. Other groups' cultural belief systems may not value asking for help or not prioritise it (see Chapter 5).

Case study

Again students reflect on why they felt unwillingness to ask for help and support:

- Sometimes, my fear of conflict prevents me from communicating effectively because I tend to keep quiet rather than express my own point of view or speak up if I feel something is incorrect.

Sometimes I cannot understand the lecturer, what he means, so I have to ask again. This is really uncomfortable for me.

- The biggest part of communication is to have to ask for help. Recently I asked for help from one of my lecturers and was really nervous to see them as I may appear stupid for just not getting it.

I initially found the online forums a little daunting as I would be admitting in writing that I did not understand something, but in reality, as my confidence grew, this was not the case and they were an excellent study tool.

Critical reflection

>> Reflect on your own approach to asking for help. For example, do you hesitate to ask because it is difficult for you?

Asking for help is critical to building your learning capacities, so don't minimise the value of this skill. However, it must be done appropriately and professionally. You need to prepare yourself – for example, by asking 'Who to ask?' and 'How to ask?' The first question often requires research. In higher education contexts, there are many sources of information: lecturers, tutors, forums, wikis, online classes, student services, learning centres, the library, faculties and departments, outreach services, the student help desk or support services offered online. It may require some investigation – including by social contact and conversation – to find the most appropriate one. It is also useful to reflect on the best way to seek help and information, as the way you ask needs to be socially and culturally fine-tuned to the particular context.

You may need to consider the actual words you will use in your verbal communication. Will you use colloquial language or jargon? Long sentences or short sentences? Will you prepare your request in advance? Do you need to practise? Will you ask directly or indirectly? How close will you stand? Physically, how and where you will ask for help (in consultation times, on a forum, using email, through an appeal if it is about a grade)? In terms of non-verbal communication, you would need to think about your gestures, facial expression, body language and whether you use direct or indirect eye contact. In terms of paralinguistics, what tone of voice, pace, volume and pitch will you use? You need to ensure that all your choices are appropriate to your context. The verbal and non-verbal ways in which you would seek help and information from your lecturer would differ from the ways in which you would ask your friends, or your employer, or a client in an aged care institution.

Participating in a group or team

The communication strategy of participating in a group or team can help you develop your confidence as well as contributing to the critical thinking and questioning that are essential in both learning and professional contexts. Team-work is crucial in workplaces like nursing or healthcare contexts.

Case study

Students reflect on their use of this strategy or practice:

- Having things like Blackboard Collaborate was extremely beneficial. The feedback, the advice I received, and the fact that I saw that people were in a similar boat with study helped me stay focused and determined.

- The online forum also did help me a lot, sharing opinions and suggestions to fellow students is a great way of learning. I have engaged in many online forums. These forums have allowed me to see how other people tackle problems and view situations, and have taught me to value others' opinions.

- I had what I thought was a lot of experience when it came to

acquiring information from digital resources. When it comes to developing my skills I realised I am not as knowledgeable as I thought. There are more ways to access information that I had no knowledge of or had access to. I found that participating in online forums was very helpful in learning due to giving and receiving advice from and to other students. I am gaining a lot of confidence and more digital literacy skills.

- A few years ago, when I was doing a social survey related to my study, I was placed in a team. My lack of self-assurance and having stage fright meant that the productivity of the entire group deteriorated.

Critical reflection

» Observe your colleagues' and peers' use of teamwork. Write down one example of a strategy that contributes to effective teamwork and one strategy that negatively affects the team's productivity.

Building your team and group capacities can not only help you to gain confi-dence in performing in education and nursing contexts, it can also help you to gain employment and/or promotion. Teamwork skills will certainly help you to accomplish academic and professional tasks more effectively and productively. However, the verbal and non-verbal behaviours and cultural beliefs underly-ing these skills also change from culture to culture, place to place and context to context. Kossen, Kiernan and Lawrence (2013) report that some individuals may feel more comfortable with teamwork while others prefer to work inde-pendently. Some groups enjoy early getting-to-know-you humour before they progress to the actual work of the meeting, handover or consultation. Some groups are more collectively orientated, while others are more individually orientated. As Chapter 5 explains, cross-cultural theory sees these differences in behaviours as cultural practices or cultural literacy. But the fact is that we often take our own behaviours and practices for granted while perceiving others' ways as different or deficit. It is important to stress that *one way is not better than the other – just different*. Chapters 2 and 9 discuss teamwork in more depth. Your nursing subjects will also draw your attention to, and develop your capacity in relation to, this critical skill.

Making social contact and conversation

Making social contact and conversation will not only increase your sources of support, but also assist in brainstorming solutions or solving problems. Your confidence in employing this practice will increase your capacity to develop networks, learning circles, mentors, friends and partners.

Case study

Again students reflect on their capacities to make social contact.

- When I came here to Australia five years ago, my communication skills were very limited. High school helped me a lot and talking to different people in English really built up my communication skills.

- I have a great support system around me including two great girls who I have met on this course. It is great to have them to talk to and ask questions; we also keep each other on track. My aunty is currently in her third year and I also have a friend who graduated last year so this is also a great avenue to receive information and get help.

- I will be working in the industry during my studies so I believe I will have plenty of help from experienced nurses when I need it.

- I didn't know anyone when I started, but I met a second-year undergraduate in the library who took me under her wing and showed me how to use the library, photocopier, Study Desk online and forums. She also added me to her study group on Facebook. I was very thankful that she took her time to show me these vital things.

Critical reflection

》 Observe your colleagues, and peers' use of this strategy. Write down three approaches you would feel comfortable using to make social contact. For example, it could be to discuss the topic of the lecture with the student beside you as you wait for the lecturer to begin. Or it could be to attend a peer support session and talk to the other students who are also attending the session.

Again, there can be differences in the ways in which individuals and groups approach this strategy, as its use needs to be socially and culturally fine-tuned to the specific context or situation. Its use depends on a very complex interplay of social and cultural factors. For example, do you need to be introduced before you are able to meet someone? Do you need to think of a suitable topic with which to start a conversation (such as the weather or a significant cultural event)? Are there 'taboo' subjects that could lead to a communication barrier, or even offence? What kinds of personal information can you use to help authenticate your status and position, which may be necessary for establishing relationships in particular cultural groups? Are there any unwritten social mores regarding this skill that would risk offending someone if you were to ignore or overlook them?

Critical practice

Critical practice can be difficult. Critical practice moves beyond your self-awareness of your own belief systems and cultural practices to include an awareness of the relationships in operation around you, which we can call *critical self-awareness*. We discussed self-awareness earlier; here we discuss critical self-awareness, or critical practice. Critical practice involves the ability to seek and give feedback about specific practices and belief systems, and an awareness of the power relationships operating in a particular context or culture.

Seeking and giving feedback are critical here. For example, teachers often give you feedback in assignments, in class and on forums. This feedback can help you to do better. Teachers want your feedback too – in student evaluations, for example – so they can improve their learning and teaching practices. In a nursing workplace, there will be performance reviews and case conferences. Seeking feedback allows you to learn more about your own practices and beliefs, as well as those of your colleagues and peers. It also allows you to check whether your understandings and interpretations about these are accurate. Asking for and giving feedback is an empowering strategy. When it is positive, it can facilitate teamwork, improve interpersonal relationships and lead to greater productivity.

Providing constructive feedback or providing negative feedback in socially and culturally appropriate ways can be difficult and risky. Yet it can be vital when it comes to being assertive, putting forward your point of view, developing flexibility, preventing stress and minimising conflict. For example, in keeping patients safe, sometimes nurses have to take their colleagues to one side and tell them that they are not doing something correctly or that the way they communicate with others is not being well received. If you were inadvertently offending someone, wouldn't it be much better if that person were to let you know?

Case study:

Student nurses reflect on situations where feedback became an important strategy in avoiding communication barriers and in enabling them to fulfil their study goals.

- The communication error I witnessed was in my class. We were learning about long bones, and our practical involved dissecting a bone from a cow. Our lecturer completely forgot to mention that the bone was from a cow. We cut the bone, and one lady was standing back. It was lucky that she realised herself that it was a cow's bone, as she followed a religion which meant that the cow was a sacred animal to her religion. It was an honest communication error for which the lecturer apologised profusely.

- I was having a conversation about my upcoming week of study and my employer was distracted by the physical environment around us – the hustle and bustle of a busy hotel. The next day he had me on the roster when I had a lab session I had to attend on campus, and we had another conversation – this time away from noise interference – to resolve the issue.

Critical reflection

>> Think about a situation where you needed to provide feedback to someone. How did you go about doing this?

If someone is offending you, then it is important for you to help to overcome this potential barrier between you by providing them with some constructive and careful feedback in a socially and culturally acceptable manner. You could use this strategy:

- Prepare what you want to say, as well as when, where and how, beforehand.
- Start with something positive and/or place yourself in their situation (be empathetic).
- Offer your specific reasons and/or explanations for why you feel offended or disagree with their view.
- Provide an alternative or state what specific action you would like them to take.

You can see the similarities between this strategy and the strategies for assertiveness described in Chapters 2 and 8.

Case study

A lecturer reflects about how she provides feedback to her students to enable them to learn more independently and to save her time when teaching large first year classes. In universities this is often called 'expectation management'.

The following protocol is one I've used when teaching courses with large numbers of students. In the first lecture I set up the 'ground rules'. This is in the context of other 'ground rules' about communicating respectfully with

peers. These are prefaced with contextual discussion about the amount of email correspondence teaching staff deal with, the nature of the teaching environment (especially collaborative learning processes) and the nature of the student–lecturer relationship (for example, we're here to help you, but you are also here to learn to help yourself/be independent learners). These include information about communications with the teaching team which should be professional and respectful, not just in terms of content.

Critical reflection

>> Do you think this kind of information is helpful or not helpful? Explain your reasons for thinking this. Provide some examples of where you either sought or gave feedback about specific practices, whether or not they achieved the solution for which you were aiming. For example, you might want to give a lecturer feedback about how marks were distributed in an assignment. Your outcome might be to have your marks increased.

Power relationships operating in a culture or context can affect your study. If you were studying social science or politics, you would be examining power relationships for the entire degree. Power is the ability to influence or control the behaviour of people. Sometimes power is seen as authority, which is the power that is perceived as legitimate by the social structure. Examples include a federal or state government, a hospital board and university council. Sometimes power can be seen as evil or unjust, and you might agree or disagree with the decisions made; however, the exercise of power is accepted as pervasive to humans as social beings. In higher education, academic staff can be seen as having more power than first-year students. As healthcare workers or nurses, you will be witnesses to power relationships both in your studies and in the clinical environment. Domestic violence – whether physical or verbal – is an expression of power. Chapter 5 discusses power from a cross-cultural viewpoint.

power relationships: relationships between individuals with differing levels of power in a specific context

Case study

I am of Aboriginal decent but due to my appearance am not recognised as such by the public. An example of discrimination was in a meeting group when one lady very openly pronounced some offensive things not only in front of me but also in front of some fellow Aboriginal students. We were all offended by the comments but chose to only discuss our feelings among ourselves afterwards. This was very unprofessional and in a patient/professional environment very inappropriate.

Critical reflection

〉〉 Identify some of the power relationships you have observed, either at university or in a clinical context.

〉〉 Reflect on when you may have experienced or witnessed discrimination.

Dynamic practices

The practices discussed in this chapter are dynamic and interdependent. The successful use of one practice often depends on the use of another and, if implemented together, they can be more effective in helping you to make a comfortable transition (Kossen, Kiernan & Lawrence, 2013). For example, observation and reflection are prerequisites for fine-tuning your capacity to make social contact within the specific context being engaged. How will you introduce yourself? Do you need to think of someone who can introduce you, for example? Likewise, participating in a group relies on your capacities to reflect and provide (appropriate) feedback about how the group is performing. The practices depend on learners' capacities to appraise not only their own cultural assumptions and expectations, but also the practices and literacies with which students need to become familiar and engage with the new context (Kossen, Kiernan & Lawrence, 2013). The capacities of learners to challenge and, where possible, to transform the unhelpful policies and practices also rely on learners' use of practices such as offering feedback, expressing disagreement and refusing a request (Kossen, Kiernan & Lawrence, 2013).

These practices are lifelong learning skills that can be applied each time you enter a new context or culture in your study or professional careers. For example, each new subject will have particular ways of communicating and operating. The practices can instil in us a resilience that enables us to apply and reapply these practices so that we are empowered to meet each new challenge as it emerges in the fast-moving and complex world in which we live. Chapter 5 will explain how these models can be applied to cross-cultural contexts.

Summary

This chapter expanded on Chapters 1 and 2 by exploring how our awareness of self shapes our capacities to adapt and make a comfortable transition to new contexts – especially higher education. The chapter asked you to identify the practices, literacies and languages that you will need to demonstrate if you are to be successful in the new context. The twin concepts of awareness of self and awareness of context were used to inform two models of transition presented at the end of the chapter. In the first model, new students need to understand their cultural background, world-views, previous educational experiences, expectations, needs and requirements as they enter the new higher education context. Thus the model visualises your transition to the new higher education as a journey, where you become familiar and engage with the new cultural practices, behaviours and literacies of the context. The second model emphasises your use of reflective, communicative and critical practices. These practices can assist you to understand the university's understandings and practices so that you are able to feel more comfortable in and be more confident about your studies. The practices are lifelong learning skills that can be applied each time you enter a new context or environment in your study or professional careers. For example, each new subject will have particular ways of communicating and operating, and you will need to make a transition every time you start studying a new subject. Moreover, the practices can instil a resilience that enables you to apply and reapply these practices so that you are able to meet each new challenge as it emerges in the fast-moving and complex world in which we live. The reflections of students were used to enrich your understandings of these transition processes.

Discussion and critical thinking questions

3.1 What transitions have you already experienced in your life – for example, moving to a new school, a new location or country, and a new culture, leaving home, starting a family?

3.2 How did you learn to become more comfortable in the new context? What strategies did you use?

3.3 Did anyone or anything support you during this transition?

3.4 What have you learnt about yourself as you reflect on making this transition?

Learning extension

Think of the clinical or work environments in which you have worked. Choose the one that was most difficult to adapt to. What made it a difficult environment for you? Was it difficult for you to learn its new languages and relationships? What do you think the organisation could have done to help you to become more comfortable? Are there lessons you have learnt from your experiences in this situation that would improve the transition experiences of others when you are in charge of a clinical environment in the future?

Further reading

Lawrence, J. (2013). Designing and evaluating an empowering online pedagogy for commencing students: A case study. *International Journal of the First Year in Higher Education*, 4(2): 49–61. This article investigates the problems experienced by first-year students transitioning to study at an Australian university. Like this chapter, it uses qualitative data from students completing a first-year communications course.

References

Korporaal, G. (2014). UQ undergraduate Ben Roberts-Smith aims to add an MBA to his VC. *The Australian*, 15 August.

Kossen, C., Kiernan, E. & Lawrence, J. (eds) (2013). *Communicating for success.* Sydney: Pearson Australia.

Lawrence, J. (2009). Two conceptual models for facilitating learners' transitions to new post-school learning contexts. In J. Field, J. Gallacher & R. Ingram (eds), *Researching transitions in lifelong learning*. New York: Routledge.

—— (2013). Designing and evaluating an empowering online pedagogy for commencing students: A case study. *International Journal of the First Year in Higher Education*, 4(2): 49–61.

Schuetze, H.G. & Slowey, M. (2000). *Higher education and lifelong learners: International perspectives on change.* London: Routledge/Falmer.

4 Communicating in academic and clinical contexts

Steve Parker and Jill Lawrence

Learning objectives

- Identify and apply the requirements and expectations about academic writing in higher education, including its purpose and structure.

- Read existing material, analyse it, assess its validity and relevance for your particular purposes, and synthesise the ideas as evidence.

- Locate appropriate sources of information and evaluate their relevance for academic purposes.

- Consistently apply the academic conventions of referencing and understand the ethical use of another's work and the complexities of avoiding plagiarism.

- Apply the appropriate elements of style and tone to your writing tasks, and demonstrate appropriate editing strategies.

- Specify the elements of effective oral presentations, and apply these presentation skills to professional nursing.

Key terms

- Academic argument

- Evidence

- Information literacy

- Main points

- Thesis statements

Introduction

One of the key practices you need to acquire and demonstrate in both academic and nursing contexts is the ability to communicate effectively. While later chapters will focus on helping you develop your capabilities in relation to cross-cultural, interpersonal, digital and organisational communication, this chapter will focus on written and oral communication in academic and clinical contexts. Communicating professionally involves developing your abilities to apply the rules and requirements of communicating in a particular context to meet an audience's purposes and needs. The chapter will first explain the role of academic writing, describing its purpose, elements and structure. This will include providing strategies to help you purposefully start your assignments and develop the main points and evidence you will need to support the argument you are building. Style and tone will also be discussed, as well as strategies that will enable you to achieve good marks for your assignments. Locating appropriate and credible evidence (part of **information literacy**) will then be discussed, as well as the importance of integrating these sources of evidence in your academic writing. The rationale for referencing, and the reasons why it is important to conform to a referencing system's conventions, will

> **information literacy:**
> a set of skills for searching for, locating, evaluating and using information

also be explored. We outline the consequences of not applying a referencing system appropriately by introducing the concepts of academic integrity, plagiarism and intellectual property. Finally, we set out the elements of effective oral presentations and apply these presentation skills to professional nursing contexts, including patient interviews and handovers. Examples and case studies are provided to assist you to apply these theoretical insights and good practices to your writing and speaking in both academic and clinical contexts. The case studies included in the chapter are students' reflections, collected as part of a research study investigating first-year students' experiences at university.

Writing academically

Purpose and context

When you write academically or professionally, you write for readers who have a set of expectations about the purpose, structure, style and tone of your writing. At university, lecturers have assumptions and expectations about academic writing. Boud (2001, cited in Kossen, Kiernan & Lawrence, 2013, p. 39) argues that 'academics have expectations, but fail to articulate them and then, potentially to make judgments about students who fail to demonstrate them'. These expectations relate to a range of writing decisions, which can include issues of:

- discipline terminology or jargon (clinical nursing language)
- structure (an essay, report, case study, reflective journal)

- grammar and expression (word choice, sentence length, punctuation)
- format (font size, margins, headings, subheadings, paragraphs)
- tone and style (colloquial or slang language, creative or emotive language, subjective or objective language, formal or informal language, use of first or third person, active or passive voice)
- sources of evidence (textbooks, subject reference lists or sources, academic texts, journal articles and databases)
- the appropriate referencing system (APA, Harvard, Oxford), direct or indirect quotes, reference lists or bibliographies
- submission decisions (hard copy, electronic, portfolio).

You need to know your subject's expectations about these writing choices.

Case study

A student reflects on how she refined her assignment decision-making during her first semester:

After failing the first assignment, I knew I had to do something different so I asked for help and found out exactly what was required for me to pass the next assignment. There are many things I have learnt from this: first, post to forums as they contain helpful information that is linked to assessment. The most important thing I learnt was to ask for help. I should have done it with Assignment 1 but I was too embarrassed and as a result I failed. This time I admitted I was unclear about what was expected of me and what I had to do. I hope gaining these valuable insights will not only help me in this subject but in my whole time at university.

Critical reflection

>> What strategies did this student use to ensure she passed her assignments?

>> Are there other strategies she could have used?

In the clinical context, you will be writing for a number of purposes and audiences. For example, you may be writing notes in patient records that describe your observations of a person's health status and your actions as a clinician in nursing them. You may also write discharge summaries for patients leaving a healthcare service, or you might develop nursing care plans that you will share with colleagues who are also caring for the patient. In all these situations, it is important to remember that a number of health professionals, as well as members of multi-disciplinary teams, routinely access your notes. Thus you need to ensure your notes are appropriate for and accessible to these multiple needs.

Academic literacy and its structural elements

A range of academic writing tasks exists. One of the most common types is writing an **academic argument**. This is a well-developed, well-structured and well-supported piece of formal writing that persuades the reader to accept your point of view. There are three main steps to developing an academic argument (see Table 4.1).

According to Kossen, Kiernan and Lawrence (2013), the first step is developing your viewpoint (your opinion/conclusion/judgement/stance) in relation to the writing task. In academic writing, this is called a thesis or **thesis statement**.

Step 2 is the generation of the reasons to support your thesis. These reasons become the **main points** supporting the thesis.

In Step 3, you need to support each main point with evidence. In academic writing, an important form of **evidence** is expert evidence (or ideas from experts, which you will find in the research literature). You acknowledge these experts by using references (usually in the text, though footnotes or endnotes are sometimes used).

These steps conform to the structure common in academic writing. Table 4.2 cross-references the steps (thesis, main points and evidence) with this structure (introduction, body and conclusion). The thesis statement and overview of main points are included in both the introduction and the conclusion. The body paragraphs each comprise one main point with its supporting evidence.

academic argument: a well-developed, well-structured and well-supported piece of formal writing that persuades the reader to your point of view

thesis statement: your viewpoint in relation to the writing task

main points: the reasons for supporting a thesis statement or the viewpoint you have taken in relation to your writing task

evidence: the information you have gathered to support each main point

TABLE 4.1 *The three main steps in academic writing*

1	The thesis	One clear, concise sentence that provides your viewpoint or argument. Your thesis should provide the reader with your opinion in relation to the question asked or topic provided.
2	Reasons supporting the thesis	These reasons become your main points, explaining and/or supporting your thesis. There is one main point per paragraph.
3	Evidence that supports and explains each main point	The evidence includes explanations or theory from experts in the subject area – the research base/theory that must be acknowledged or referenced and examples to apply and extend the theory and/or referenced explanation you are using to support your main points.

Source: Adapted from Kossen, Kiernan & Lawrence (2013)

TABLE 4.2 *Cross-referencing steps with academic structure*

STEPS	STRUCTURE
Thesis statement Overview of main points	Introduction
A series of paragraphs, each explaining one main point that is supported by evidence	Body
Thesis statement Review of main points	Conclusion

Source: Adapted from Kossen, Kiernan & Lawrence (2013)

- The *introduction* provides background information that engages the reader's interest, the thesis statement and an overview of the main points.
- The *body* is made up of a series of paragraphs, with each body paragraph explaining one main point. The body paragraph begins with a first sentence (often called the topic sentence), which states the main point of the paragraph and links it back to the thesis. The remainder of the paragraph provides the evidence supporting this main point.
- The *conclusion* provides an overview of the main points, draws conclusions and strengthens the thesis. No new information is included. Generally, the conclusion does not contain references, because references are considered to be evidence – and evidence does not belong in the conclusion (Kossen, Kiernan & Lawrence, 2013).

When you are reading textbooks and journal articles, you will see that academics use this same structure when they write. Understanding this structure can help you to more efficiently find the main points and evidence you need to support your arguments when you are writing your assignments.

A writing strategy

Understanding the structure of academic writing and its built-in repetition will save you time and energy, as well as help you to focus on what you have to do to complete your academic writing task. The writing process can be made easier by breaking it up into smaller, more manageable steps or activities that you can tick off as you go. According to Kossen, Kiernan and Lawrence (2013), these include finding out about assignment expectations, analysing the writing task, generating a draft plan and beginning the writing process.

Find out the assignment expectations

Having a clear understanding of the task of the assignment, its weighting and how it will be marked is a time-saving strategy because it designates how much effort you will then need to put into each part of the writing process. At university, these sources of information include marking or criteria sheets, rubrics, any sample assignments, lecture and tutorial information, learning centre support, resident fellow support if you are in college, the library, fellow students and your study group or learning circle.

Analyse the task

There are three factors to consider in analysing what you have to do: the task, the content and the limits imposed by the task (see Table 4.3).

TABLE 4.3 *Analysis of the task*

FACTOR	DEFINITION	EXAMPLES
Content	Tells you what the assignment is about	What is the subject or topic area the question wants to know about?
Task	Tells you what you have to do	Usually a verb tells you what to do. Do you have to analyse, describe, define, explain, etc.?
Limits	Tells you how to limit the scope or content of the question	Tells you what area to focus on; defines the topic further. Is there a particular timeframe, place, book, etc.?

Source: Adapted from Nash (2011) and Klossen, Kiernan & Lawrence (2013)

Analysing the verb or task (what you have to do) leads you to make decisions that determine how you will approach the content. It also gives you clues as to the form or structure of your writing. Some lecturers are not explicit about the meaning of task words, so it is always useful to ask what a task word means. Some of the more common task words are: *analyse, argue, compare and contrast, define, describe* and *evaluate*. This process of analysing the task helps you understand it and focus your research, and will ensure you answer the question that has been asked.

There is a great deal of information on the internet about the meaning of task words. Investigate the meanings of task words and write down a definition of each to assist you when you are beginning to write an academic argument.

LEARNING ACTIVITY

Generate a draft plan

In generating your draft plan, you need to develop a thesis and the main supporting points.

Develop your thesis

You can try using the wording of the actual task or question, but make sure to turn it into a stance. For example, the question might ask you to analyse a clinical aspect of hand hygiene in a particular context of your choice. Your thesis then might be something like, 'Using alcohol rubs as a form of hand hygiene is more effective than ordinary hand washing in preventing infection from spreading on cruise ships.' Another approach is to read the task, then rewrite it. Use words with which you are familiar, then write your own version. When you are writing your assignment, ensure you keep your thesis close by, frequently checking it to make sure you are focused on the assignment question. You need to be aware that your thesis might change as you engage more with the question or topic, and refine it further.

Generate a thesis statement from the following question. You need to write one concise sentence that will reflect your answer to the question and drive your academic argument. When it is completed, check your thesis with a peer for feedback.

Select a common wound type (e.g. diabetic foot ulceration, pressure ulcer, leg ulcer, fungating wound, dehisced surgical wound) and analyse how you would provide care for it in your role as a qualified nurse. It may help to reflect on a patient with this type of wound for whom you have cared.

A possible thesis could be:

The role of a qualified nurse in treating a patient with a pressure ulcer includes the provision of wound hygiene and infection prevention.

Note that the patient you choose would become the example you would use as evidence in each of your body paragraphs.

Apply the process you used above to one of your writing tasks this semester.

Develop your main points

Either brainstorm main points from your thesis or research for main points using the recommended texts for the subject. A mind or concept map (see Figure 4.1) can be useful because the relationships between the thesis and the main points can be clarified.

Conclusion:
Overview of main
points plus thesis

Main point

Introduction:
Overview of main
points plus thesis

Question
(leads to thesis)

Main point:
Evidence =
• references
• examples
• explanation

Main point

Main point

Main point

FIGURE
4.1

Mind map planning
Source: Adapted from Kossen, Kiernan & Lawrence (2013).

Identify the thesis statement and main points in this article abstract (or summary), then insert them into a mind map. Check your mind map with a peer or colleague.

LEARNING
ACTIVITY

Healthcare workers' hands are the most common vehicles for the transmission of healthcare-associated pathogens from patient to patient and within the healthcare environment. Hand hygiene is the leading measure for preventing the spread of antimicrobial resistance and reducing healthcare-associated infections (HCAIs), but healthcare worker compliance with optimal practices remains low in most settings.

This paper reviews factors influencing hand hygiene compliance, the impact of hand hygiene promotion on healthcare-associated pathogen cross-transmission and infection rates, and challenging issues related to the universal adoption of alcohol-based hand rub as a critical system change for successful promotion.

Available evidence highlights the fact that multimodal intervention strategies lead to improved hand hygiene and a reduction in HCAI. However, further research is needed to evaluate the relative efficacy of each strategy component and to identify the most successful interventions, particularly in settings with limited resources.

The main objective of the First Global Patient Safety Challenge, launched by the World Health Organization (WHO), is to achieve an improvement in hand hygiene practices worldwide with the ultimate goal of promoting a strong patient safety culture. We also report considerations and solutions resulting from the implementation of the multimodal strategy proposed in the WHO *Guidelines on Hand Hygiene in Healthcare*. (Allegranzi & Pittet, 2010, p. 305)

Find the evidence

You can support your main points with different forms of evidence, which can include theory, research or the research base, and explanation and examples.

Theory is an explanation of why something happens or is important (see Chapter 2). For example, hand washing is important in healthcare because of the theory explaining the chain of infection, and therefore its use in stopping the spread of infection. For example, in a nursing course, beginning nurses not only need to know that they must wash their hands but also *why*. So students learn Semmelweis's germ theory (see Hanninen, Farago & Monos, 1983). Semmelweis discovered that the incidence of fever could be reduced significantly by the use of hand disinfection in clinics. He proposed the practice of washing with chlorinated lime solutions while working in a Vienna general hospital, where doctors' wards had three times the mortality of midwives' wards.

The meanings attached to theory can change depending on the context. For example, in daily life people refer to unproven ideas and speculation as *theories*. These sorts of theories provide informal knowledge about the world. Alternatively, formal theories like Semmelweis's germ theory are more rigorously tested, and therefore have greater authority and credibility (Kossen, Kiernan & Lawrence, 2013). In the sciences, a theory is rigorously tested and is measurable – which means it can be used to explain an experiment or to find out whether something is true and accurate, and can be repeated.

In the academic context, theory is important because it provides a perspective on why we do things or think in certain ways. It is partly why some professions have moved their training from their places of practice or work to the university context, as the theoretical understanding that university provides increases professional standing. For example, nursing moved from the hospitals to higher education in Australia some 30 years ago.

The *research base* often includes theory, and is referred to as the 'literature', a 'review of the research' or a 'literature review'. It describes research or information already conducted in a particular area and written about by experts in the field. It is the academic convention that if you want to conduct research in an area, you must first consult the research base or literature that already exists in the area. This helps you establish what is known and not known about a given topic. It also shows readers you are familiar with the significant and up-to-date knowledge relevant to your topic. Incorporating the ideas/explanations of subject experts in your paragraphs supports your argument as a form of evidence to explain/support your main points. In fact, many of your textbooks are literature reviews as they report and summarise the findings of research that other people have conducted. Ultimately, referring to the research base in your topic area helps you to establish the credibility of your argument, as it provides expert support (or evidence) to reinforce what you are claiming. Referencing this research base is essential in underpinning the academic credibility. It is not enough to provide this research evidence; you need to say where it came from and when it was printed. Referencing is discussed later in the chapter.

Explanations and examples are also a form of evidence used to support the main point. Examples can be used to explain theory or research. In the writing task, if you are asked to analyse a patient's disease or given a case study, the examples will stem from or be linked to the thesis statement. For instance, if the thesis is limited to the circulatory system, then the examples need to be linked to (limited to) the circulation system as well.

The more specific the example, the more convincing it will be. Instead of 'scientists can be effective when communicating with the public', a more specific example would be 'Karl Kruszelnicki is an Australian scientist who builds rapport with his audience by giving simple explanations and using humour' (Kossen, Kiernan & Lawrence, 2013). Instead of the relatively brief example 'the clinical team would need to seek permission', a more specific example would be 'a member of the clinical team would need to seek the patient's permission before revealing any information the patient had disclosed about their personal circumstances' (Kossen, Kiernan & Lawrence, 2013). Providing examples also makes your writing richer, and enhances its emotional impact. This is important for motivating the reader to engage with your argument.

Explanations and/or examples help you apply or link the theory or research to practice. If you just include the theory, then your writing may be too descriptive because you haven't linked the theory or research. For example, by applying Semmelweis's germ theory to the infection chain on a cruise ship, you are explaining the link between theory and practice, which means your reader has a better understanding of the theory. Explanation needs to relate to either the research evidence or theory used. Through using explanation, the main idea is elaborated and its meaning explained further. For example, the theory of hand hygiene can be explained by providing information about how the infection spreads in a particular context, like an aged care facility or a pre-school. It is also useful to think of the power of examples in assisting you to understand theory. For instance, lecturers use specific examples to help you understand the more complex concepts and theories they discuss.

Have the examples used in this chapter been useful for helping you to improve your academic writing? Explain how.

Begin the writing process

Having collected and developed your thesis, main points and evidence, it is now time to begin writing your paragraphs. Each main point corresponds to one paragraph, and the paragraph's first sentence should explain this main point. It is important to understand that the main point is *neither a quote (either direct or indirect) nor an example*. This is because examples and referenced material comprise the evidence that supports the main point. The rest of the paragraph integrates the evidence, including any theory, research and explanation/examples. The next learning activity provides one example of how these elements can be structured in the body of the paragraph.

LEARNING ACTIVITY

The following paragraph was written in response to an assignment question that asked: 'Discuss a clinical aspect of hand washing, making sure to include a context.' The thesis chosen was, 'Hand rubbing with a waterless, alcohol-based, rub-in cleanser is more effective than using a regular hand-washing technique with soap and water.'

Your task is to identify the main point and the different forms of evidence used to support the main point, including any theory, research and explanation/examples. Also check whether the referencing is consistently used and conforms to a particular referencing system.

> The side effects of rubbing with a waterless alcohol-based, rub-in cleanser are rarer than the side effects caused by using soap and water. Hand washing with plain soap can cause skin dryness, cracking and irritation, especially if living in a cold, dry climate (Rhinehart & Friedman, 1999). Some people, for example, find their dermatitis is exacerbated in winter especially if washing with harsh soaps. However the cleanser-rub has far fewer side effects. According to Widmer (2000, p. 140) a 'database of 3500 HCWs generated over 10 years did not identify a single case of documented allergy to the commercial alcohol compound in use, which resulted in an estimated incidence density <1:35,000 person-years'. Widmer (2000) also maintains that allergies to alcohol are rare and could only be caused by emollients and other compounds added to the alcohol. Many organisations now provide their employees with waterless, alcohol-based rub-in cleansers, which points to the efficiency and lack of side effects being experienced with these types of products. It is important for nurses to be informed about the side effects of all products, especially those that are used frequently.

The next section discusses strategies you can use to locate the evidence you need to support your thesis statements.

Information literacy

Information literacy is the ability to search for, locate, evaluate and use the information needed (Eisenberg, 2008).

Searching and locating sources of information to use as evidence

Information literacy relates to your ability to locate the evidence to support the argument you are writing. If you are a student, your university library is the most appropriate source of information about this literacy. So, rather than provide information here that is not contextualised to your particular higher education institution, we encourage you to investigate your own library site. Most libraries provide online sources of information as well as classes (on campus and online) that have been devised to assist you to develop the skills of information literacy. This is a crucial aspect of academic literacy, and it is important that you empower yourself in its use.

Case study

Students' reflections reveal the library practices that students found surprising:

- The most surprising thing I have learnt about the library is the virtual availability and the ability for books to be posted out wherever you are; great flexibility. The role the library plays within the university is in learning development, whether that be self-directed (access information through books, e-articles) or group study sessions or workshop groups.

- I have found the library tutorials to be very helpful. I have been quite nervous to use the online library as I have found them quite difficult to use in the past, however after watching the tutorials and going through a few activities I am feeling more confident about using the library. The tutorials are so helpful in showing how to find a particular article, book or video. I will definitely be referring back to these in the future! The library is definitely of extreme importance in university study and it is hugely helpful when referencing as you can be sure that information you find is genuine, as opposed to what can be found on the internet!

- One of the most surprising things I have discovered about libraries in university study is just how vital they are to academic work! No more 'just Googling' opinions and following them! I also have been surprised at how thoroughly searching a library for a certain topic can greatly change the way you actually view your assignment. What may have seemed a clear-cut answer *before* you started researching now looks much more complicated once you have actually taken the time to search the library.

- One of the most important aspects for me about using libraries is how it forces you to organise what you're doing before actually getting your information. To enter in correct keywords and get useable articles, you first have to have a general idea of what your topic is, be able to expand it into various keywords and phrases, and be able to decide which articles are relevant and which articles are not, even before you start the real researching! So libraries play a much bigger part in achieving success in uni than I ever gave them credit for in the past!

- I have studied previously and was surprised by the number of tutorials available to assist. I found that the tips and hints for researching, as well as searching in the library catalogue were of the most benefit. I've been overwhelmed at the sheer volume and different types of information, but feel much more confident now that I can perform succinct and relevant searches when required. Finally, my biggest surprise is the availability of library staff to provide assistance. I suppose from my high school days with a grumpy 'shushing' librarian, I have always had some trepidation in asking for help. I now know that there is no need to hesitate with the librarians only a phone call or an email away.

One of the most surprising things I found out about the university library is how accessible everything the library has to offer is for online and external students too. I love the fact that I can access databases 24/7 – given I work shiftwork, my study hours are a little varied. I feel like a great deal of effort has gone into making you feel as though you have the same opportunity for information as students who can physically attend the library. It is essential to have academic studies to support your own statements or theories as part of academic writing. Now all I have to do is practise navigating by myself.

Critical reflection

>> Describe three ways in which the library can be useful for your studies.

>> List three strategies you will use to improve your information literacy this semester.

>> Investigate your university or higher education website to locate the type of help your institution offers about finding appropriate sources of information.

Evaluating sources of information

Another aspect of information literacy is the capacity to evaluate sources of information. Again, you will find information, tutorials and podcasts on your library site to assist you to evaluate sources of information. A first step is to ask a series of questions about the authority/credibility of the author(s) and the journal or publisher, as well as its currency and accuracy:

Does the source of information have authority?

- What can you find out about the authors?
- What are the authors' qualifications and experience?
- Are they recognised in their field?
- Have they written anything else?
- Are there any linked biographical statements, resumes or other background about the authors?
- Are the authors associated with a society, institution or professional organisation?
- Have they been given a grant to do their research?

- What can you find out about the journal/publisher?
- What is the journal?
- Who is the publisher?
- Is the journal peer reviewed (which means the articles are assessed anonymously by experts in the field)?
- Is it a credible source?
- Is it an official site or private/business site?
- What is the purpose – to sell/persuade/inform?

Is the article current?

- When was the material written, submitted and accepted?
- What is the date of publication?
- Are the references current/up to date?
- When was the site last updated or revised?

Is the article accurate?

- Is the information reliable and free from error? How can you tell?
- What is the source of the information – a research study, a literature review, a personal story?
- Can you verify the information?
- Is there in-text referencing?
- Is it supported by a bibliography or list of references? Are these linked?
- If it is research, was it funded? By whom?
- Are details given about the participants, ethics, etc.?
- Has the information been through an editorial and refereeing process, or a quality assurance process?
- For controversial topics, is the presentation biased (one-sided) or balanced (with both pro and con viewpoints)?

Case study

Students reflect on their development of this aspect of information literacy:

- During the process of evaluating the article's authority, currency and accuracy, I went back to notes that I had from doing a STEPS course to gain university entry. I have always struggled with finding information to support my arguments as I find I become overwhelmed with articles and which is the best to use. When I found the article that

I chose on hand hygiene in a child care setting I had just spent hours going through the university library database without finding anything that seemed to fit. I ended up finding my article through Google, which I was hesitant to use, however as it was an article from NCAC (National Childcare Accreditation Council Inc.). I decided to stick with it as I know from my work in child care that this is a reputable source of information regarding child care policies and procedures. I then looked to who it was written by and what sort of experience she has in this field and how recent it was written. After reviewing all of this I decided it was a credible source of information for this activity.

- In order to assess my article on its authority, currency and accuracy, I firstly wrote down a list of questions (that I actually noted down from this week's lecture) for each characteristic. After that, I searched for the answers on

each aspect in several different areas. I started firstly within the article itself, as there was a little information on the author included. Then I got info from the database such as when it was published, who published it, when it was reviewed, etc. Then I did both a database search and an internet search to discover more about what the author had written and what his qualifications were. Then I did a search on the journal in which the article was published to discover the academic standing, reputation and credibility of the actual journal.

Critical reflection

>> Describe the strategies the students used to check whether their information was credible.

Referencing academic sources

Why reference?

The university context is an individualised, hierarchical culture where research and knowledge are valued. You cannot get an academic job at a university, for example, unless you have started to develop your own research profile.

Another powerful motivator for referencing correctly and accurately comes from the idea of 'intellectual property'. Intellectual property takes us back to the notion that in the Western academic world ideas belong to people. Ideas are the property of the person who thought them up, and to use them without indicating this is considered to be stealing their ideas.

It is productive, however, to understand that using words and ideas from credible sources and indicating where they came from adds significantly to the information's *value and credibility*. Kossen, Kiernan and Lawrence (2013) argue that referencing demonstrates that you:

- have consulted the research literature
- have used an expert research base to support your main points
- know how important referencing is in the university's academic culture
- understand that readers/markers can check the original source to make sure that you are not misrepresenting it.

Thus plagiarism and academic integrity are intertwined: stealing ideas is plagiarism and plagiarism constitutes academic misconduct. Acts of plagiarism are therefore seen by universities as acts of misconduct for which you can be penalised, so developing study practices and writing skills that allow you to avoid plagiarism is essential. Plagiarism can occur when you use another person's work without full and clear referencing and acknowledgement, and when you are presenting another student's work as your own. This belief system is not the case for all cultures, however. In many cultures (mainly collective cultures), the use of another's ideas and words is considered to constitute recognition of their esteem and a reference is not required. However, you are studying in a Western academic culture where referencing is mandatory.

What to reference

Understanding which information to reference can be confusing for beginners. The rule is that you need to reference all information you use from other sources. For example, the following sources of information must be referenced in academic writing:

- all quotations from all sources
- any statistics or case studies to which you refer
- any unusual facts or findings from a source
- any definitions, as a definition has no credibility unless it is defined by an expert
- any information you paraphrase or summarise from a source
- any idea, theory or information from a source.

How to reference

Basically, there are two steps to referencing. First, in the body of the assignment, you insert in-text references where you have used the ideas or words of others (see Table 4.4).

TABLE 4.4 *Referencing in the assignment body*

STEP 1: IN THE BODY USE IN-TEXT REFERENCING (IN APA STYLE)	
Either	**Or**
Use the exact words (a direct quote):	Paraphrase or use the idea (an indirect quote):
The Nursing Code of Conduct from the Australian Nursing and Midwifery Council (ANMC) is Code of Conduct Statement 7, which states that 'nurses support the health, wellbeing and informed decision-making of people requiring or receiving care' (ANMC, 2008, p. 4).	The Nursing Code of Conduct from the Australian Nursing and Midwifery Council (ANMC) Code of Conduct Statement 7 states that nurses need to consider how they can support their patient's capacity to make informed decisions about their care (ANMC, 2008).

Source: Adapted from Kossen, Kiernan & Lawrence (2013)

TABLE 4.5 *Referencing at the end of the assignment*

STEP 2: IN THE LIST OF REFERENCES (IN APA STYLE)

Australian Nursing and Midwifery Council. (2008). *Code of Professional Conduct for Nurses in Australia.* Sydney: Nursing and Midwifery Board of Australia.

Source: Adapted from Kossen, Kiernan & Lawrence (2013)

Second, at the end of the assignment, you insert the full bibliographic reference to the source of the information used in a reference list (see Table 4.5).

This is called the 'References' or 'Reference list'. It includes all the sources of information cited (or included) in the body of the assignment. If the reference list includes all these references as well as others you have read but not actually cited in the body of the assignment, then it is called a 'Bibliography'. In the APA and Harvard referencing systems, this list is written in alphabetical order by author and date.

Case study

A student's reflective conversation with their online tutor reveals the complexity involved in becoming familiar with referencing systems and conventions:

Student query:
I found the journal article on the university's library search then followed it to the original site. While we can read it on the library site, I have referenced it to its original site which requires a subscription to view it. Is this correct for referencing or should I have referenced it to the library site? I'm not sure I followed all the instructions available.

Tutor reply:
You're pretty close with your citation and I'll give you some direction in a moment. First, I will tackle your question about the DOI or URL details. If what you have looked at is an electronic version of what would otherwise be in print, then you do not absolutely *have* to include the details from the database or website. However, for the purposes of this week's activity it is good practice to do so to make sure you know how to include that. In your assessment work, if you provide all other details correctly for a journal article or book chapter, you are unlikely to be asked for the DOI or URL. Of course, if it is an e-journal that *only* exists online, then you would definitely include the web address.

Now, to your citation – you need to italicise the *journal name* and journal *volume number*, as per the USQ library guide to APA:

Sullivan, E. (2003). Off with her nails. *Journal of PeriAnesthesia Nursing*, *18*(6), 417–418. doi:10.1016/j. jopan.2003.09.002.

Critical reflection

》》 Critically assess your referencing skills, and if you are losing marks for referencing in your assessment items consult your library's referencing site and refine your skills.

Your academic referencing literacy will take time to develop – it doesn't happen overnight. Kossen, Kiernan and Lawrence (2013) provide the following referencing tips:

- Never begin the paragraph with a quotation. Quotations should be used to support, not replace, the main point of the paragraph.
- Reference sooner rather than later in the paragraph, as this adds to the credibility and authority of the information/evidence you are providing in a paragraph. Consider referencing in the second or third sentence of the paragraph. The first sentence is, of course, the main point and written in your own words.
- Do not place an in-text reference at the end of the paragraph, and assume that the reader will realise that all the information in the paragraph came from that source. You need to reference immediately after you have cited the information.
- Following on from the previous point, if the evidence in the paragraph does originate from the one source, then indicate this by integrating the referencing with a lead-in phrase like: 'Thomas (2014) puts forward the following argument' or 'Da Vinci (2014) nominated the following strategies'.
- Look up the particular referencing system you are using to see how large, direct quotes should be presented.
- When you are citing/referencing a source who the author has referenced in their work, you show this by writing it as, 'Perrin, 2000 cited in Hughes, 2014, p. 22' (where Hughes, the author of the article you are reading, has cited the work of Perrin). Only Hughes is included in the reference list.
- It is more sophisticated to paraphrase than to use direct citations. Use direct quotations only when you cannot put the ideas into your own words as effectively – for example, where the quotation has very 'wise' wording that really 'speaks' to what you want to say, or where they are the exact words of some auspicious authority.
- Never compose the paragraph as a string of quotes: quote, quote, quote. This signifies that your own voice (through your selection of the thesis and main points) is not heard.
- Always define your key terms, but not by referring to an ordinary dictionary or Wikipedia. This helps you avoid the fallacy of an 'appeal to authority'.
- Never give a definition or state 'research says' without providing a reference, otherwise it will constitute the fallacy of an 'appeal to authority'.
- Never use a generalisation without an in-text reference; otherwise it will be a 'faulty generalisation'.

Editing your academic writing

Editing for style and tone

In addition to its referencing expectations, academic writing has further rules. There are also requirements about the *way*, or *how*, we write, which is referred to as 'style and tone'. Style relates to the writer's choice of words and structure, while tone is the feeling conveyed by the writer's style (Nash, 2011, cited in Kossen, Kiernan & Lawrence, 2013). The style and tone preferred in academic writing are formal and objective.

How can you ensure your style and tone are appropriate? First, observe how we write for you in academic sources like database articles and texts.

Read the following abstract:

Hand hygiene compliance in healthcare is a new concept in Vietnam, and it has now become a national priority to improve healthcare workers' practices according to current recommendations. In this study, hand hygiene compliance among healthcare workers was audited following an intervention including education and the introduction of alcohol-based hand rub during the first hospital-wide hand hygiene campaign conducted at a 2100-bed tertiary hospital in Hue, Vietnam. Recourse to alcohol-based hand rub was more frequent than hand washing with plain soap and water (83% and 17%, respectively; P = .0001). Hand hygiene compliance averaged 47% (1,310 actions/2,813 opportunities; 95% confidence interval [CI]: 45%-48%) with markedly different rates among departments, ranging from 5% to 69% (P = .0001). (Salmon et al., 2014, p. 178)

What do you notice about the style and tone used? Are there creative and/or emotional words and phrases included? Is it first, second or third person? What punctuation is used?

Notice how textbooks (such as this one) sometimes use first person (I, me, mine, myself, we, us, our, ourselves) and second person (you, your, yourself) pronouns, while some of the more formal articles and readings, like the one in the learning activity, use third person (he, she, they, her, his, their, itself, oneself, themselves) pronouns. Academic writing can be both formal and informal. Textbooks can be more informal because the writers want to make the information easier for students to read. We want you to feel we are on your side. However, articles from prestigious journals are written in a more objective and formal tone and style. Such academic writing strives to be objective, as reason and rationality are highly valued in the university culture and academic writing normally reflects this. For example, the use of just one factor – first, second or third person pronouns – can change the style and tone of the writing. First person (I, we, our) reveals the writer's personal thoughts. It is informal and subjective. Second person (you) is informal, appeals to the reader's personal view or feelings and assumes they don't want an informed and researched view. The writer's presence is obvious. It is informal and subjective. Third person (they, nurses) means the writers' thoughts and opinions are removed from the information and research evidence is used to inform readers. It is important to note, however, that different readers, markers and journals may vary from these general rules. It is essential to check with the person or organisation for which you are writing to confirm what the expectations are.

There are a number of other factors that can influence your choice of style and tone. The following list from Kossen, Kiernan and Lawrence (2013) tells you *what not to do* when writing academically in an academic context:

- An unnecessary repetition of words can detract from your writing, making it look awkward – for example, 'comprehend and understand', 'large depth' and 'simple and humble'.
- Avoid emotive/creative language. Rationality is valued in higher education. Such words as 'ideal', 'merely', 'even', 'of course', 'proof', 'truth', 'extremely' and 'still' appeal to the reader's heart, not their rationality.
- Avoid 'absolute' terms. The use of words like 'all', 'only', 'never' and 'every' is not valid (for example, not 'all' students enjoy university study).
- Avoid exclamation marks. These create an emotive response in the reader (think of your average email or text, where their use often indicates sarcasm on behalf of the writer).
- Generally, avoid abbreviations in formal assignments. Abbreviations such as 'e.g.', 'i.e.' and etc.' are not appropriate when you are writing a formal, objective assignment. These abbreviations are not a good 'look' in academic writing.
- Avoid colloquial expressions and slang terms. Academic writing takes itself seriously. Notice that when I include a 'colloquial' word in this chapter, I enclose it in single inverted commas. In the previous point I wrote 'look' to indicate that I know that 'look' is a colloquial term and that it really has no place in academic writing.

Analyse the tone and style in the following excerpts. How does the writer convey this tone and style? Why did the writer choose this particular style and tone? What was the purpose and where might you find these pieces of writing (on a poster, on the internet, in a poetry book)?

LEARNING ACTIVITY

a   I like washing my hands as I like the water coating my hands, the feel of the soap on my fingers and the fizzy suds as they bubble up from the soap. I concentrate on thinking mindfully as I try to hold my hands under the cool, clear, running water for the two minutes that the tattered posters plastered on the mirror in front of the basin recommend.

b　As you touch people, surfaces and objects throughout the day, you accumulate germs on your hands. In turn, you can infect yourself with these germs by touching your eyes, nose or mouth. Although it is impossible to keep your hands germ-free, washing your hands frequently can help limit the transfer of bacteria, viruses and other microbes. Always wash your hands before:

> ❭ preparing food or eating
> ❭ treating wounds, giving medicine or caring for a sick or injured person
> ❭ inserting or removing contact lenses.

c　Medical hand hygiene pertains to the hygiene practices related to the administration of medicine and medical care that prevents or minimises disease and the spreading of disease. The main medical purpose of washing hands is to cleanse the hands of pathogens (including bacteria or viruses) and chemicals, which can cause personal harm or disease. This is especially important for people who handle food or work in the medical field, but it is also an important practice for the general public.

d　Hands:
> Calloused, darkened by sun, weathered by drought and despair
> Crimson tipped, indulged, pampered and nourished daily
> Tiny, imprinted in vivid yellow, transported from kindy and fixed to the kitchen fridge
> Symbols, icons even, of experience, of connection!

Editing the final draft

Editing is a very important step in the academic writing process. In higher education it is the step that will prevent you from losing valuable marks. In academic writing, lecturers often include a checklist to assist you. The marking criteria or rubrics may also provide information about tone and style in the form of the task criteria about grammar, spelling, expression and accurate referencing (all of which need careful editing and all of which non-verbally provide the reader with information about your choices of tone and style).

A key factor of editing is the requirement related to pacing yourself. It is hard to edit carefully when you have left the task to the last minute. The first step is to edit it carefully yourself. A second strategy is to ask someone else to edit your assignment for you. These editors may include a friend or sibling or parent, or a member of your study group or learning circle. Differentiate between editing for content and editing for grammar, spelling, punctuation and structure. It is also useful to read a sentence out loud if you are not sure whether it makes sense. Be mindful in checking tone and style, word choice, sentence length, paragraph length, thesis statement, topic sentences, introductions and conclusions, presentation, punctuation, setting out, expression and spelling.

Writing in clinical contexts

Writing in clinical contexts can be challenging because of the diversity of reasons for writing, the variety of people for whom you are writing and the different tasks that require writing. Some examples of writing include:

- documenting patient care in medical records (paper or electronic)
- writing instructions for patient information
- documenting procedures
- producing discharge summaries
- developing nursing care plans for patients
- writing and responding to emails.

There are many more, and each writing activity has its own 'rules' to follow. In addition, to make the situation even more complex, different organisations may have their own styles and guidelines for writing in various situations and documents.

The best way of dealing with this is to work from some general principles of good writing and apply them in whatever situation you need to write for. Paul and Elder (2007) offer some excellent guidance on how to write well, which needs to be applied to writing in a clinical context. The following is based on their work, which you can follow up in more detail in the reference provided.

When you approach a writing task in a clinical context, there are a number of very useful questions you can ask about your writing. Ask these questions as you write anything and improve your writing as you answer them for yourself. Here are the questions taken directly from Paul and Elder (2007). Underneath each question are some comments for you to think about when specifically writing in a clinical context:

- Why am I writing this? What is my purpose? What do I need the reader to come away with?

  This is a very important question because you will need to write differently for different purposes. For example, if you are writing a nursing note in a patient record, you will need to follow the conventions of the organisation for which you work, and think about how you convey what you need to in concise, accurate, comprehensive language. If you are writing a patient discharge summary that is to accompany a patient when they later visit their GP, the letter will need to convey a brief but accurate summary of all the nursing care provided and the care required following the hospital stay.

● Is there some part of what I have written that I don't really understand? Perhaps I am repeating what I have heard people say without ever having thought through what it exactly means.

> If you don't know the exact meaning of what you write, then you need to be very careful – especially if someone is relying on the information or instructions you are providing to implement care for a patient or client. If you are a student or the language you are communicating in is not your primary language, you will need to take extra care that you understand what you are writing. The best approach is to not write what you don't understand. Find out the meaning of terms you don't understand or check with someone who can explain them to you. When you understand, then you can write with confidence.

● If something I have written is vague, how can I make it clearer or more precise?

> If you write something vague, it allows lots of room for misinterpretation because your reader will tend to insert their own understanding into what you have written. It can take quite a bit of practice, but writing in as precise a manner as possible is important in a professional context.

● Do I understand the meaning of the key words I have used, or do I need to look them up in a dictionary?

> Once again, this is really important if you are a student, if the language you are communicating in is not your native language, or if you are new to a practice area. If you are not sure *you* understand the meaning of the words, you may be using them incorrectly and conveying the wrong meaning. This can have very serious consequences if people are making decisions or taking action in response to what you write.

● Am I using any words in special or unusual ways? Have I explained special meanings to the reader?

> All language occurs in a context and, if understanding is to occur, you must use language that is mutually understood. In addition, professional language can often have precise meanings that may not be exactly the same as general usage. So if you are not sure that you are using words correctly, look them up in a dictionary. For professional words, use a dictionary that is specialised, such as a dictionary for nurses or a medical dictionary.

● Am I sure that what I have said is accurate? Do I need to qualify anything?

> Written language can easily be misunderstood, especially when you don't know who might be reading what you write. And in professional contexts,

accuracy is a key standard for which you need to aim. Make sure you check facts by going back and reading documents such as nursing notes, doctors' orders or what someone has said in handover. Your accuracy (or lack of it) may seriously affect someone else.

- Am I clear about my main point when I write clinically, and why I think it is important?

  As you write, keep asking yourself whether you are sticking to the point and purpose of your writing. Try to remove anything not relevant to your purpose.

- Do I know what clinical task or question my paragraph is answering?

  All sorts of writing occurs in a clinical context – for example, nursing notes, reports, emails and discharge planning summaries. Some of these can be lengthy, and it is easy to lose sight of the overall purpose of what you are writing. If you are writing a lengthy document, ask yourself whether the section or paragraph you are writing has a purpose. It may be asking the questions: *What is the evidence for what I am claiming?* or *What examples illustrate my main point?* It is often useful to look at something you are writing and convert it into a question or a response to a question. This helps keep your writing clear and on track.

- Do I need to spend more time investigating my clinical topic or issue? Do I need more information?

  Whenever you write, it is important to know that you have considered all the relevant information, that you have checked it for accuracy and that you are clear in your own mind that you have a good grasp of the big picture. Sometimes, it is appropriate to ask for more time to write something so that you can explore the issue further. It is better to delay your writing and provide good quality than to rush and discover later that you leapt to a judgement that was incorrect or dangerous.

A final suggestion when writing in a clinical context is to have someone you trust check what you have written if you are unsure about it. This is a strategy that is used by even very experienced writers. It is particularly useful if you are writing anything when you are emotionally involved in the topic or situation. Humans are inevitably involved emotionally – it is not possible to be emotionless. The whole point of seeking a second opinion is to ensure objectivity when needed. Many issues related to good writing communication can be resolved by this simple strategy, so be courageous enough to share your writing with others.

Oral communication

Formal oral and written communication modes have many similarities: they each need to develop an argument (thesis, main points and evidence) and are structured in the same ways (introduction, body and conclusion). Everything we have discussed above can be applied to oral communication, including the questions to ask when writing. This section looks at some of the specific principles that apply to oral communication.

General principles of oral communication

There are literally thousands of books on communication and how to communicate well. We don't want to cover the same ground, so here we offer you some powerful principles of communication to keep in mind as you speak and listen to others.

Principle #1: People respond to our communication in the way they understand the world

As we grow and experience life, we all create a map of reality in our minds about how the world works and the meaning of words and behaviours that form part of communication. So when two people communicate with each other, they interpret everything according to their map. Words that may mean one thing to one person may mean something entirely different to another. The same goes for non-verbal behaviours. Lots of eye contact might make one person feel very uncomfortable, while for someone else it may be the very thing that makes them feel as though they are being listened to.

This means that an essential part of communication is to learn as much as we can about the other person's way of understanding the world. Chapters 2 and 3 provide some practical strategies to assist you to understand others' world-views or ways of knowing. But the most effective way of doing this is to reflect on your own belief systems in this situation, learn to listen well, ask probing questions and carefully observe how others respond to you. You can then adapt your communication so that it 'fits' with the other person's understanding and your communication is likely to be much more successful. This requires a deep respect for the other person's experience and understanding, and well-formed skills of listening and flexibility.

Principle #2: The meaning of any communication is determined by the context of communication

Sometimes people argue about the meaning of what they say by appealing to dictionary definitions without realising that meaning can change depending on the situation in which we are communicating. It's very important to take the context of communication into account when listening and speaking. The command 'Get help!' might mean something entirely different in a hospital when a nurse discovers a person collapsed on the floor compared with a conversation with a friend who is having trouble with a boyfriend, and you are suggesting that they get some support from a counsellor. The context of any communication must *always* be taken into account.

Principle #3: Communication is like breathing

Breathing has a rhythm to it – we breathe in, pause very briefly and breathe out. This happens over and over again. Breathing in is like the listening phase of communicating. We focus our attention on what the other person is saying. Then, just as there is a brief pause before breathing out, there should be a brief pause before we speak so that we can reflect on what we have heard and respond appropriately. Then, as we breathe out, we speak in response to the other person. In the same way that you cannot breathe in and breathe out at the same time, it is impossible to listen and speak at the same time. Too often, we tend to be thinking inside our heads about what we are going to say next rather than focusing completely on the other person as they speak to us. This often leads to communication that is misunderstood or comes across as though we haven't genuinely listened. To communicate well, we need to practise this rhythmic approach to communicating so that we truly connect with others in genuine, respectful dialogue.

Oral presentations at university (or anywhere)

Let's move now to two specific places in which oral communication occurs. The first of these is when you are asked to present orally as part of your learning at university. The second is when you communicate orally in a clinical context.

Orally presenting at university is sometimes required as part of assessment or classroom activity. I'm sure you have listened to many presentations already during your life experience, and many of them probably could have been more engaging, shorter or more interesting. A quick search on Google for 'why most presentations suck' will provide you with lots of information about how poor most presentations are. Here are some principles for ensuring that your presentations are effective and engaging.

Principle #1: Have a clear idea of the main point you wish to make in your presentation

In the same way that writing needs to have a clear thesis or conclusion, so does an oral presentation. Everything we have outlined above about writing applies here as well.

Principle #2: Decide on a maximum of three sub-points to support your main point

Oral presentations should, as a rule, not be more than about 20 minutes long (of course, this doesn't include your university lectures, which are often much longer). This means you need to be concise in what you say and to think carefully about the most relevant ideas needed to support your main conclusion. You need to continually think about what is absolutely necessary to include and draw on the most powerful and persuasive evidence in support of your presentation.

Principle #3: Find out who your audience is, where the presentation will take place and what resources are available to you

The more you know about your audience and where you will be making the presentation, the more you can adapt your presentation to the audience and design what you do using the technology that might be available. Knowing what the room is like also helps you design an appropriate experience for your audience, and can reduce the anxiety that is often associated with turning up to a new room and needing to be orientated.

Principle #4: Question the common assumption that you have to do all the talking

Presentations can take a lot of forms, and the most interesting ones are those that are innovative and include some form of audience engagement. So think about things like group discussions, question and answer times, using video and audience contribution. A lot of this will depend on *why* you are presenting. If it is part of an assessment at university, then you will need to check the assessment requirements and discuss what you are planning with your lecturer.

The following principles are provided to you on the assumption that you will use some form of presentation software to support what you say (although you should question whether you always need to – some presentations are better without slides). The most popular software is Microsoft PowerPoint, but there are others available.

Principle #5: Presentation slides are for your audience – not you

Many presenters use their slides as 'notes' for them to remember what they need to say. But slides are meant to illustrate and support what you are saying during your presentation. One of the worst mistakes you can make is to read from your slides. Slides need to be carefully designed to be engaging, powerful, visual hooks that convey key points you are making. Some of the following principles will help you design better slides.

Principle #6: Use pictures rather than words on slides

There isn't much that is worse than sitting through a presentation where slide after slide is full of text. Wherever possible, use a well-designed picture to illustrate what you are saying, and remove unnecessary words from your slides.

Principle #7: Use the 10–20–30 rule whenever possible

A common set of guidelines for presentations is the 10–20–30 rule: use no more than 10 slides, present for a maximum of 20 minutes and, when using text, use a font that is not less than 30 points. In addition to these points, if you do use text on your slides, try to use no more than three dot points per slide and no more than three words per dot point. These guidelines can be challenging to implement, but they will make your presentations more engaging.

Principle #8: Practise

Practising your presentation a few times before delivering it can help you deal with anxiety (because you gain confidence the more you practise), help to identify changes you might need to make and (if you practise with another person) obtain feedback on how your presentation comes across.

Principle #9: You don't have to be perfect

If you are like most people, you may make some mistakes. It is important to remember that you don't have to be perfect – in fact, perfection is an unattainable goal. This is not an excuse for lazy preparation or poor design of your presentation. It is a reminder that we are all human and we all make mistakes – even if we have done lots of practice. Most audiences like to know that you are one of them – or perhaps that you have made mistakes like them. It helps to add credibility to what you say. Even though you may do everything possible to prepare and deliver your presentation, things sometimes go wrong. That's okay – it happens to everyone. It is worth having some alternative ways of presenting your material if you are using technology of some sort, just in case anything goes wrong. And if you are just starting out doing public presentations, you need to allow yourself the opportunity to make mistakes and learn from them. If you follow the above principles, even if you do make mistakes, your presentation will be effective and professional.

Take a look at this brief video about good presentation slide design: <http://youtu.be/eLGLtnRopJM>.
   How will you change your presentations in future to overcome some of these problems?

Oral communication in the clinical context

Communicating in clinical contexts is complex. The general principles of communication described in the earlier discussion about writing in clinical contexts are equally important in these contexts. Healthcare is increasingly recognised as needing high-level interprofessional communication. With clinicians working in different specialty areas and collaborating with other disciplines, the need for good communication is paramount if healthcare is going to succeed in delivering successful outcomes for patients and clients.

One of the most interesting developments in the area of clinical communication is a program called TeamSTEPPS™, developed by the US Agency for Healthcare Research and Quality. TeamSTEPPS™ is 'an evidence-based teamwork system to improve communication and teamwork skills' (AHRQ, 2011). The system provides a number of key communication strategies for clinicians to use as they work in healthcare teams. Even if the TeamSTEPPS™ approach is not in place across a health service or team, individuals can make use of the strategies in their own professional communication. For now, here are just some of the strategies available that you might think about using as part of your communication in clinical practice. They are all taken from the *TeamSTEPPS™ Pocket Guide* (AHRQ, 2006).

ISBAR

ISBAR (the official acronym of the TeamSTEPPS program) is 'a technique for communicating critical information that requires immediate attention and action concerning a patient's condition' (AHRQ, 2006, p. 28). Even if a team member does not know about this format of communicating important information about a patient, you can use it to structure your own communication. See Chapter 2 for a more in-depth discussion of ISBAR.

Call-Out

Call-Out is a 'Strategy used to communicate important or critical information' (AHRQ, 2006, p. 29) between team members. You have probably seen this strategy used on TV shows in emergency departments, when the leader of a team calls out something like, 'Pulse?' and the reply comes from a nurse, '96!' Or, 'Blood pressure?' with a response, '110/60!' According to the *TeamSTEPPS™ Pocket Guide* (AHRQ, 2006, p. 29), the Call-Out strategy:

- informs all team members simultaneously (about information) during emergent situations
- helps team members anticipate next steps
- helps team members be aware that it is important to direct everything to a specific individual, who is responsible for carrying out the task of leading the Call-Out process.

In most emergency situations in clinical organisations, there will be a similar process, so when you work in a clinical area, you should find out what the process is there so that you are familiar with it.

Check-Back

Check-Back is a process of employing 'closed-loop communication to ensure that information conveyed by the sender is understood by the receiver as intended' (AHRQ, 2006, p. 30).

Check-Back is the TeamSTEPPS™ process by which a person who communicates information then confirms (or corrects) your understanding. In the TeamSTEPPS™ program, this procedure is explicitly agreed upon so whenever any information or directions are communicated, both parties engage in the process; this means there is absolutely no doubt that the information or direction is understood. For example, a doctor may give an order such as 'Give 15 mgs of morphine IV'. The nurse would respond, '15 mgs morphine IV'. The doctor would then say, 'That's correct'. So the communication 'loop' between the doctor and nurse is closed off and the instructions are known to have been communicated clearly.

The *TeamSTEPPS™ Pocket Guide* (p. 30) summarises the steps in the Check-Back strategy in this way:

1 The sender initiates the message.
2 The receiver accepts the message and provides feedback.
3 The sender double-checks to ensure the message was received.

This is a very useful communication strategy. Even if you work in a place where there is no explicit agreement to use this approach, you can still ask others to repeat back to you whatever information or directions you provide so that you are sure they understand your message.

There are many more strategies and tools in the TeamSTEPPS™ approach. We encourage you to explore TeamSTEPPS™ further. Many health services are training their staff in this approach, with positive outcomes. Whatever you do to develop your communication skills in clinical practice will be worth it, and will improve your job satisfaction and the outcomes for your patients and clients.

Summary

This chapter introduced the literacies related to communicating in written and oral contexts in higher education and in clinical situations. The role of academic writing was examined, including its purpose, elements and structure. Strategies to assist you to purposefully start your assignments and develop the main points and evidence you need to support your arguments were also outlined. Locating appropriate and credible evidence (information literacy) was then discussed as well as the importance of integrating sources of evidence in your academic writing. The rationale for referencing and the reasons why it is important to conform to the conventions of a referencing system were also explored. Finally, the chapter specified the elements of presenting effective oral presentations and their application to professional nursing contexts, including patient interviews and handovers.

Discussion and critical thinking questions

4.1 What are the specific rules or requirements that higher education institutions expect students to be able to demonstrate in relation to academic writing?

4.2 Why is the thesis statement so important in academic writing?

4.3 Why are style and tone important in academic and in clinical writing?

4.4 What are the key principles you can integrate when giving powerful presentations?

Learning extension

Think about the knowledge you have gained about writing and speaking in specific contexts.

- Choose a writing or speaking task you found difficult to complete. Why was it difficult for you?
- Think about the skills and strategies you will now use when you begin such a task. Describe how these strategies will increase your confidence to complete the task effectively.
- What strategies will you use to check whether or not you did complete the task successfully?
- What lessons could you pass on to others that would improve their writing or speaking experiences in the future?

Further reading

Agency for Healthcare Research and Quality (US) (AHRQ) (2006). *TeamSTEPPS™ pocket guide*. Retrieved 20 January 2014 from <http://www.ahrq.gov/professionals/education/curriculum-tools/teamstepps/instructor/essentials/pocketguide.pdf>.

Hazelwood, Z. & Shakespeare-Finch, J. (2010). *Let's talk: Communication for health professionals*. Sydney: Pearson Australia.

References

Agency for Healthcare Research and Quality (US) (AHRQ) (2006). *TeamSTEPPS™ pocket guide*. Retrieved 20 January 2014 from <http://www.ahrq.gov/professionals/education/curriculum-tools/teamstepps/instructor/essentials/pocketguide.pdf>.

—— (2011). TeamSTEPPS™. Retrieved 20 January 2015 from <http://teamstepps.ahrq.gov>.

Allegranzi, B. & Pittet, D. (2010). Role of hand hygiene in healthcare-associated infection prevention. *Journal of Hospital Infection*, 73(4): 305–15.

Eisenberg, M.B. (2008). Information literacy: Essential skills for the information age. *DESIDOC Journal of Library & Information Technology*, 28(2): 39–47.

Hanninen, O., Farago, M. & Monos, E. (1983). Ignaz Philipp Semmelweis, the prophet of bacteriology. *Infection Control*, 4(5): 367–70.

Kossen, C., Kiernan, E. & Lawrence, J. (2013). *Communicating for success*. Sydney: Pearson Australia.

Nash, G.J. (2011). *A guide to writing argumentative essays*. Melbourne: John Wiley & Sons.

Paul, R. & Elder, L. (2007). *The thinker's guide to how to write a paragraph*. Foundation for Critical Thinking, Tomales, CA.

Rhinehart, E. & Friedman, M.M. (1999). *Infection control in home care*. Maryland: Aspen/Wolters Kluwer, Amsterdam.

Salmon, S., McLaws, M.-L., Truong, A.T., Nguyen, V.H. & Pittet, D. (2014). Healthcare workers' hand contamination levels and antibacterial efficacy of different hand hygiene methods used in a Vietnamese hospital. *American Journal of Infection Control*, 42(2): 178–81.

Widmer, A.F. (2000). Replace hand washing with use of a waterless alcohol hand rub? *Clinical Infectious Diseases*, 31(1): 136–43.

5 Building transcultural skills for professional contexts

Coralie Graham and Jill Lawrence

Learning objectives

- Specify your understandings of culture and apply these understandings to cultural difference and diversity.

- Understand how cultural misunderstanding can arise.

- Develop cultural competence to ensure cultural safety for all client populations.

- Examine the nuances of culturally appropriate care in a range of client populations.

- Apply the two models introduced in Chapter 3 to your clinical placement experiences.

Key term

- Culture

Introduction

> I acknowledge the traditional owners on whose land I walk, I work and I live.
> I pay my respects to Elders past and present.

This is an Indigenous protocol and an illustration of intercultural respect. In the Australian context, this protocol means acknowledging that there were about 180 language nations that resided on this land before 'Australia' was 'discovered'. I pay respect to this protocol by including it on my emails, and using it at the start of my lectures, or when presenting workshops and giving speeches. I acknowledge the protocol because it recognises the cultural, institutional, social, economic and global contexts within which we all live and work, interacting with many different local and global communities and **cultures**. Every time we communicate, we do so through our own cultural understandings, just as the people with whom we are communicating interpret what we are communicating through their

culture: what people do every day: how they behave, speak, relate and make things

own cultural lens. This chapter investigates how our cultural understandings influence our communication. It argues that to become effective professionals, we need to understand our own culture and how it affects our communication, and manage the cultural and language differences that are pivotal to living and working in the twenty-first century. The chapter also provides strategies that will help us to communicate effectively with the diverse cultural groups and sub-groups we encounter in our study and professional lives.

It is important to be aware that our personalities also influence how we communicate. Chapter 6 explains how personality or individual differences can affect communication. Across cultures too there are many similarities in experiences around life, work, change and death. It is therefore also important to appreciate that cultures often have more in common than they do differences.

Defining culture

The concept of culture has a range of everyday and technical uses and meanings. Lankshear et al. (1997, cited in Kossen, Kiernan & Lawrence, 2013) describe these different meanings:

- culture as artefacts (e.g. 'early Aboriginal culture is displayed at the museum')
- culture as visible displays (e.g. 'the cultural dances of the Pacific')
- culture as ethnic or racial identity (e.g. 'there are 60 cultures represented at the University of Southern Queensland')
- culture as 'class' (e.g. 'they have culture and style')
- culture as 'high' or 'low', or 'elite' (e.g. 'the opera is an example of high culture')
- culture as exotic or different (e.g. 'Indigenous culture is "raw"')
- culture as explicit rather than implicit (i.e. you can see it, touch it, hear it, taste it and perhaps smell it).

These definitions of culture are 'narrow' in that they associate culture with material objects (dance, drama, diet and dress), visible displays (ceremonies and festivals) and other tangible features, such as language or dialect. They understand that culture is what you can see, touch, hear, smell and taste. These narrow definitions imply that culture belongs to others, and that 'we' don't have culture; they infer that our behaviour is 'normal and natural', and it is the cultural behaviours of others that are different.

It is not that these narrow definitions of culture are incorrect; rather, this chapter argues that there are wider, more productive ways of thinking about culture that are more appropriate in our contemporary world. This wider concept of culture suggests that we all have culture – that culture is reflected in our everyday activities, relationships and social processes, our values, beliefs, norms, customs, possessions, rules and codes, and our assumptions about life. Shor (1993, p. 30, cited in Lankshear et al., 1997) argues that 'culture is what ordinary people do every day, how they behave, speak, relate and make things. Everyone has and makes culture…culture is the speech and behaviour of everyday life'. For example, while eating is seen as a biological process, the foods we eat and the ways in which we prepare and consume them are examples of cultural activities. Eating with chopsticks, knives and forks, with our hands, around a table, in front of the television, in a hotel, or at a fast food restaurant or a dumpling stall are all examples of cultural practices (Kossen, Kiernan & Lawrence, 2013). In Lawrence (2014), a nursing student notes that:

> My culture and Australian culture have many differences. First, in Australia they eat at the table with knife and fork but in my country we eat by hand and from one plate.

As Chapters 2 and 3 have already discussed, this wider concept of culture is confirmed by its presence in many different theoretical perspectives. In anthropology or ethnography, culture is a central concept. Words and phrases like 'way of knowing' and 'world-view' are also key to the theoretical perspectives of social science and critical theory (see Kossen, Kiernan & Lawrence, 2013). Communication theory uses words like 'perception' (outlined in Chapter 2), 'interpersonal communication' (outlined in Chapter 6) and 'organisational communication' (discussed in Chapter 7).

The wider concept of culture can also be applied to more specific groups within societies. Each of us belongs to a range of cultural groups and sub-groups – a family group or groups, social groups, friendship groups, work groups, sporting groups, religious groups, gender groups and so on.

Think of your groups of friends. Are there differences in the ways the members of each group relate to or communicate with each other?

We are simultaneously members of many cultural groups, each of which may have different cultural practices and/or share common practices. We are also members of the cultures that are emerging from globalisation – for example, Facebook, Twitter and other social media (see Chapter 7).

There is also a national culture or identity. Australia is a multicultural country. Aboriginal and Torres Strait Islander peoples have been here continuously for 60 000 years (Hazelwood & Shakespeare-Finch, 2010), but everyone else is an immigrant of less than 250 years' heritage. Australia has a high level of first- and second-generation immigrants. In 2006, for example, 25 per cent of Australians were born overseas (ABS, 2006, cited in Hazelwood & Shakespeare-Finch, 2010). However, the numbers of migrants and Aboriginal and Torres Strait Islander people vary across Australia. For example, only 1.6 per cent of the South Australian population identify as Aboriginal and Torres Strait Islander people compared with 27.8 per cent of people in the Northern Territory (ABS, 2006, cited in Hazelwood & Shakespeare-Finch, 2010). International students are surprised by the diversity of cultures they encounter at university (Lawrence, 2014):

> I found it shocking that Australia is a multicultural country as Australia has got mixed cultures and is not limited to one specific culture.

> When I came to Australia I was very surprised to see that Australia is a multicultural country. Many people came from different countries with different languages, different beliefs, different values and different cultures.

Despite this diversity, Western ideas of communication are the norm in Australia. For example, English is used as the standard language, written communication is valued (particularly in legal matters) and the accessibility of ideas (especially through the internet) is a taken-for-granted notion reflecting the individualised Western way of communicating. The next section discusses how cultural differences operate in our professional lives in academic, nursing and healthcare contexts.

Cultural difference

Identifying how cultural difference can arise is important if we are to act professionally in all the contexts with which we engage. If we have not been exposed to different cultures and to different ways of understanding and knowing, we might not understand the uncertainty posed by wider concepts of culture. Here we introduce the ideas that each cultural group communicates using specific verbal and non-verbal behaviours and that the same act can have different meanings in different cultures. We also describe the ways individually and collectively orientated cultures differ in their approaches to life, and acknowledge the cultural differences inherent in the way men and women communicate.

Verbal and non-verbal differences

Each cultural group communicates using specific verbal and non-verbal behaviours. According to Kossen, Kiernan and Lawrence (2013), these include greeting people, eye contact, personal space, silence, dress, use of time, taking turns in conversations and speaking. Our body language, our gestures, the way we eat and our 'naming' practices can differ between cultural groups. When we greet people, for instance, we might shake hands or bow, or envelop the newcomer in a bear hug, or kiss them on either cheek or exchange business cards (Kossen, Kiernan & Lawrence, 2013). The most appropriate behaviour is finely tuned to the particular cultural context we are in at the time. Likewise, the use of eye contact differs from culture to culture. In white Australian culture, direct eye contact is interpreted as a sign of confidence and honesty. In some Asian and African cultures, direct eye contact is a sign of disrespect, or possibly challenge. Calling people who are in a more senior position or older by their given name is seen as disrespectful. Lawrence (2014) presents the following anecdote from a nursing student:

> At higher education boys and girls are together and they can call their teacher by their first name and they speak with me like their friends. However, in my country when we call our teachers we say 'teacher' and when we answer a question we should stand.

The same act can have different meanings in different cultures. For example, speaking in a quiet voice is a sign of respect in some cultures, but a sign of concern or shyness in others. Waiting for others to finish their sentence is a sign of courtesy in some cultures but is not valued and accorded little respect in others – for example, Australian culture. These differences relate to our behaviours (our cultural practices). In discussing how health practices can differ between cultural groups, Hazelwood and Shakespeare-Finch (2010) provide examples related to the Xhosa people in South Africa and Aboriginal and Torres Strait Islander peoples in Australia. The Xhosa people train people who hear voices to be healers and look up to their prowess in this regard while in Western medicine people who hear voices are perceived as being in need of medication. In their traditional law, Aboriginal and Torres Strait Islander peoples perceive mental illness as external to the individual and perhaps the result of an offence against traditional law. Health professionals need to be aware that such differences exist and should be mindful of them in the clinical context.

Individualist and collectivist cultural differences

Hofstede (2001, 2014) was a seminal cultural researcher who identified four dimensions to cultural difference: power distance, uncertainty avoidance, masculinity-femininity and individualist-collectivist. Power distance refers to the ways people in various cultures react to status differences and social power. Uncertainty avoidance refers to how cultures adapt to change and cope with uncertainty. Masculinity-femininity refers to the way cultures prefer assertiveness and achievement (masculinity) or nurturance and social support (femininity).

This section focuses on individualist and collectivist cultural differences, which are particularly relevant to assumptions or ways of thinking that are intrinsic to both Western academic and healthcare cultures. For example, differences between individualist and collectivist cultures emerge in relation to referencing conventions. In Western academic culture, there is an understanding that ideas (and words) belong to individual people. Therefore, it is important to acknowledge the owner of the idea (words) explicitly in an in-text reference. Not to do so is labelled plagiarism and is considered stealing or cheating. Some other cultures do not share this view; in these cultures, it is respectful if you quote the idea but not the source. Another way in which these differences can cause confusion is in relation to setting out the complete bibliographic reference. In individualist cultures, it is the individual's name that is expressed first – for example, I write my name as Jill Elizabeth Lawrence. However, in collective cultures the surname (family name) is written first – for example, Yang Hwei-Jen. So an international student coming from a collective culture may have difficulty deciding which name to reference as the surname in a bibliographic reference.

According to Hofstede (2001, 2014) individualist cultures, such as Australia, New Zealand, Canada, Britain and the United States, are more likely to pursue individual activities and agendas than to contribute to the success and well-being of the larger group. In these cultures, a high degree of independence/self-reliance/individual problem-solving is valued (Hofstede, 2001). It is reflected in the use of individual desks in education, the use of individual cars rather than public transport (despite the negative effects of urban sprawl, air pollution and highway/parking congestion), the notion of individual owner-ship, and the concept of control over one's personal property. Privacy is impor-tant, and life choices – such as those concerning marriage, jobs and children's names – tend to be made individually.

In a collectivist culture, people tend to view themselves as members of groups (families, work units, tribes or clans, and nations) and usually consid-er the needs of the group to be more important than the needs of individuals. There is an emphasis on collective well-being (the well-being of a group) and social harmony (Hofstede, 2001). Most Asian cultures (for example, China) and some European and African cultures tend to be collectivist. While in in-dividualist cultures people are permitted to speak out and challenge ideas be-ing put forward by other group members (Hofstede, 2001), collectivist cultures tend to reach decisions through careful consensus, and there is a tendency to avoid conflict and speaking out against issues. Given the emphasis placed on harmony and conformity, collectivist cultures tend to communicate less direct-ly and much more politely than individualist cultures, in which communication tends to be more direct or 'to the point'. An example of this kind of indirectness is a library sign in South Korea that reads, 'There is much laughter and fun in our trees and park outside'. A cultural translation in many English-speaking countries would be, 'Silence in the library'. This shows how cultural norms re-lating to manners can require a substantial shift in the way we think about and approach communication, as there can be large differences in people's cultural sensibilities.

Collectivist and individualist approaches are not better or worse than each other; rather, they have different underlying taken-for-granted assumptions about life, which can in turn provide us with different perspectives. These ways of behaving or knowing can be beneficial in some situations. For example, people from collectivist backgrounds can be well suited to teamwork and avert-ing group conflict. Yet the tolerance of group conflict in individualist cultures promotes competition between ideas, which can also help to produce effective outcomes.

It is also important to understand that our cultural orientation can some-times inhibit our use of productive communication strategies. Scott, Ciarro-chi and Deane (2004) suggest that people with strong individualist views have smaller social support networks, are less likely to seek support for personal problems and have less skill in dealing with emotional well-being than others whose views are not so strong. In an Australian rural setting, this may mean that supposedly self-reliant farmers or teenagers may be less likely to ask for help when experiencing suicidal thoughts or if they are overwhelmed by adversity. That is why organisations as varied as Beyondblue and Men's Sheds Australia explicitly talk about joining groups and asking for help.

Cultural stereotyping

There is considerable intellectual discussion about the way in which cultural stereotypes develop. Socialisation, early carer influence and the media are implicated in the way we perceive and categorise people who are from a particular group. McGarty, Yzerbyt and Spears (2002) note that shared stereotyping is useful (but often not accurate) in understanding or predicting the behaviour of a particular group. Hofstede's (2001, 2014) value orientations predicting the way in which members of a particular cultural group may act or communicate are a type of stereotyping. So there always needs to be an understanding that there will be individual differences within any cultural group. As students and healthcare professionals, we need to examine our own socialised cultural stereotypes to ensure that any personal negative stereotypical views do not negatively impact on either the quality of care we are able to provide or the cultural safety of our patients. It is vital that nurses suspend any negative judgements of any people under their care (Andrews & Boyle, 2002).

Within broader national cultures, there are smaller subcultural groups called microcultures, with their own power structures, rituals, beliefs and rules. The next section applies the more general cultural understanding perspectives outlined above to the healthcare culture.

Healthcare culture

Healthcare culture is one example that has clearly defined hierarchy, behavioural differences, distinct style of dress (uniform), a unique language and a number of rules about social interactions that differ significantly from the national culture in which they are embedded. For nursing students, the new healthcare microculture can present some unique challenges as they negotiate the typically unwritten rules of the new culture. Suominen, Krovatin and Ketola (1997) observe that there is very little written about healthcare culture, and there continues to be very little formal study of this area. It is wise to have some 'pre-travel' or preliminary information from others familiar with the new culture. This is where your lecturers and clinical preceptors can assist you. Using the practices outlined in Chapters 2 and 3 can also be helpful here.

Negotiating healthcare culture

Historically, the shift from hospital to higher education nursing education has involved the role of the registered nurse requiring a greater knowledge base and a more autonomous and respected healthcare practitioner. There has also been an increase in the amount of respect and autonomy accorded the role of the registered nurse in Australia and other developed countries. From a cultural perspective, the power distance or hierarchical structure within healthcare settings is much more structured and more clearly defined than it is in the wider Australian community. Similarly, the need for clear lines of authority and the call to minimise ambiguity in all communication to safeguard patient safety means that communication within healthcare settings tends to be much more direct than it is in the broader population.

The non-verbal element of personal space is another area of significant difference between broader Australian culture and healthcare culture. For example, when providing treatment, nurses need to be physically closer to patients than is usual outside a healthcare setting. Although healthcare professionals are accustomed to close physical and often intimate personal interactions, we still need to gain consent from our patients and explain what we are planning to do and why it is important. The need for this consideration is even greater in cultural groups where higher levels of personal modesty are the cultural norm (see later in this chapter for a discussion of particular cultural groups).

Negotiating unfamiliar language

When first entering a healthcare context or workplace, it is important to recognise that there will be a new or unfamiliar language. To further challenge you in the new healthcare culture, the new complex language is filled with multiple acronyms and commonly used healthcare jargon. This language use can lead to semantic barriers (see Chapter 2), and generate difficulties in your interactions with healthcare professionals. Therefore, it is vital that students studying nursing have a foundational knowledge of basic healthcare terminology prior to their first clinical placement as part of their undergraduate nursing degree.

A number of healthcare acronyms are used as common language in a healthcare setting. To complicate matters, there are also many commonly used healthcare acronyms related to medication and treatment that are specific to specialised areas. Many are Latin, and their full meanings not intuitive – particularly for students whose first language is not Latin-based like English. Examples include mane (morning), nocté (night), prn (when required), stat (immediately), tds (three times a day) – there are many others.

The Australian Commission on Safety and Quality in Health Care (ACSQHC, 2006) has published a list of acceptable commonly used abbreviations/acronyms and identified a number of abbreviations that have caused adverse patient events due to the acronym being mistaken for something different. For example, the abbreviation/acronym CA can be written to represent carbohydrate, (cancer) antigen, cancer, cardiac arrest or community-acquired. ACSQHC recommends writing the full medical term in patient charts, followed by its acronym, in the first instance to ensure patient safety.

Despite these recommendations, it is common in healthcare settings to hear sentences constructed almost entirely of healthcare jargon and acronyms. The following sentence would be easily understood by most healthcare professionals, but might terrify a patient.:

> When the MVA gets back from MRI he should have his PRN stat, and then set up an IV with a PCA and check his MCS on his micro-urine – I think he has a UTI.

A short explanation of what the healthcare professional is saying would alleviate considerable stress if he knew that what was being said meant:

> When the man who had the motor vehicle accident gets back from having his x-ray, he should have his medication immediately, then the equipment needs to be set up for a drip with a pain-management system for the patient to use. The pathologist should then be contacted to check on a test, as I think the patient may have a urinary tract infection.

As is immediately obvious, the version with acronyms is not only time efficient but very specific, and saves considerable time in a healthcare setting, but can cause significant unnecessary patient stress if not explained.

It is important to recognise that once we have been immersed in healthcare culture for even a short period of time, we often forget that the language we are using is not easily understood by people outside this environment. This is where you can use the practices delineated in Chapter 3 and help patients to understand the language used. It is wise to place yourself in your patient's shoes and remember how little *you* understood before you started nursing. This allows you to help your patients and explain their healthcare in lay or everyday terms.

Cross-cultural communication in healthcare teams

With increases in the numbers of graduating nurses born outside Australia, being part of a multicultural healthcare team is now standard in most workplaces. In 2011, 33 per cent of nurses, 56 per cent of GPs and 47 per cent of specialists in Australian were born overseas (ABS, 2013). This significant, continuing increase of doctors and nurses from other countries enriches the workplace; however, it can also present many communication challenges in the healthcare environment. The increase in English language proficiency requirements for a registered nurse in Australia (AHPRA, 2014) has reduced spoken-language errors in healthcare environments. Given that less than 7–10 per cent of the meaning of communication is from verbal communication (or the words alone), there is still a high potential for miscommunication when there are cultural differences in team membership in a healthcare setting.

Case study

Bai is a 28-year-old female second-year nursing student from Taiwan who is starting her clinical placement on a busy Australian metropolitan hospital surgical ward. She has completed all the preliminary paperwork prior to commencing her placement, has arrived at the ward on time as arranged and has asked at the desk for her preceptor, Ruth (the Nurse Unit Manager). She is aware there are other students from the same university also starting their placement, but does not know them other than by sight, as they are Australian domestic students and Bai tends to stay in her group of Taiwanese students when she is on campus. The ward clerk tells Bai that Ruth is busy and will soon see her. The other Australian students arrive shortly afterwards and are given the

same message. A few minutes later, a nurse hurries up to where they are all waiting, smiles and makes a hand signal indicating to Bai and her fellow students that they should come with her. Bai follows her, but the Australian students stay where they are, chatting. When the nurse realises that Bai is following her, she snaps at her to get back to where she was told to wait. Confused and upset, Bai returns to where she was and waits with the others.

In this case study, Bai has misread a common Australian hand signal that means to wait for the moment as an almost identical Taiwanese hand signal that means to come. Although the other students didn't follow, it was inappropriate for her to ask her preceptor out of respect, so Bai followed her as she thought she was meant to. When Ruth told her in an annoyed way to get back to where she was told to wait, Bai was confused as she did not know what she had done incorrectly.

Critical reflection

>> What other non-verbal gestures are you aware of that have ambiguous meanings cross-culturally?

>> How might cross-cultural differences in personal space impact on the way people behave? And how does it make you feel if people stand too close or not close enough?

Case study

Radha, a 23-year-old Indian nursing student, is waiting on the same ward with her Australian fellow students. Ruth arrives and tells them all to follow her, which they do. Ruth gives them each four patient charts and tells them to read the charts and 'take a gander' at their patients. Confused by what she is meant to do, Radha reads the charts then goes back to the desk and stands to wait for Ruth's next instruction. After half an hour, Ruth finds Radha standing and waiting. She seems annoyed, and comments to a colleague that Radha is lazy.

Ruth's perception that Radha is lazy is based on her seeing that Radha has failed to follow Ruth's instructions. On the other hand, Radha did not understand what 'take a gander' meant, so once she had finished reading the charts, she returned respectfully to wait to be told what to do next. Waiting respectfully for an authority figure to provide further instructions is valued in Indian culture. The Australian students, who had understood that they were to go and meet their four patients, were seen as showing initiative, which is valued in Australian culture.

Critical reflection

>> Would you ask for clarification if you were in this situation? What aspects of medical culture might prevent you from asking?

>> Can you think of some other commonly used Australian colloquial terms that might create misunderstanding?

Case study

Ravi is a 30-year-old nursing student from Nepal. He has come to see his lecturer at university to ask advice about his assignment during the designated time when the lecturer has said she is available. When Ravi arrives at the lecturer's door, it is closed. He waits respectfully for several minutes, then leaves without knocking.

Ravi has not knocked on the lecturer's door as, from his cultural perspective, it would be very rude to disturb a person in a senior position. This is an example of dissimilarity in power distance between Australian and Nepalese culture, where Australia scores quite low on this domain, indicating there is greater equality in organisations when compared with Nepalese cultural higher scores, which indicate a marked and strongly observed hierarchy in all aspects of society. Similarly, Ravi's expectation (that he would be heavily directed by those senior to him) has the potential to create misunderstandings in an Australian context where initiative and independence are expected.

Similarly, in Radha's situation in the previous case study, Ruth's expectation was that, having read the charts, the students would meet the patients and see what needed to be done for them.

In both Ravi and Radha's cases, the clinical preceptor's impression will possibly be that the students are lazy and lack initiative, rather than understanding that they are being respectful of the preceptor's more senior position. It is vital that those in positions of responsibility in student supervision are aware of cultural differences, and acknowledge that these differences can lead to misunderstandings during clinical placement. For example, the clinical preceptor's awareness that students who come from a high power distance culture might interpret actions differently means supervisors will need to clearly outline the appropriate practices expected during clinical placements.

Another potential source of misunderstanding stemming from differences in power distance is the reluctance of many patients to ask questions and to seek clarification. Patients and their families are less likely to ask questions about conditions and treatments than they would be in the broader Australian community because of the greater hierarchical and power differences in healthcare settings. To this can be added the vulnerability of all unwell patients. The disparity and potential for miscommunication are amplified when patients or family are from a higher power distance culture (Hofstede, 2014), where questioning those with perceived higher power is inappropriate. It is important to encourage your patients and ensure that they feel safe in asking questions about their care.

Because of differences in power distance, Ravi and Radha are very unlikely to ask for clarification if they do not understand the colloquial expressions used. This is also common with patients from all backgrounds, who do not understand healthcare jargon and acronyms. Again, amplified power distance differences in the healthcare culture mean patients and family members would be less likely to ask for clarification. Nurses need to be mindful about the possibilities for misunderstandings in their communication with patients and families, and ensure that they are comfortable and given opportunities to ask questions and seek clarification.

Case study

Susan, an Australian nursing student, is on clinical placement in a busy surgical ward. The condition of one of her patients has begun to deteriorate. The registered nurse asks Susan to phone Dr G, the specialist, and ask him to come to the ward to check on her patient. Susan is aware of Dr G's reputation for rudeness, and knows he does not like students being on the ward. She is very anxious about phoning him, and hesitates.

Critical reflection

» How might you feel in this situation?

» What could you do to reduce your anxiety, but still meet your patient's needs?

» How do you cope where there are such big power differences?

Susan's case further illustrates the power differences that exist in medical culture. Outside medical culture, such power differences are less clearly defined, and might even be able to be avoided completely. In a case such as this, where patient needs are paramount, healthcare staff need to develop strategies for communicating and effectively advocating for their patients. It is also important to note that patients and healthcare staff who have grown up in a collectivist culture are likely to have a stronger sense of family commitment than is typical in the broader Australian community. Although Australian healthcare staff, patients and family members care deeply about family members, they are more likely to negotiate caring responsibilities with others. Being from a collective culture may mean healthcare staff are unavailable to work due to family commitments, or patients' relatives may insist on staying with an ill family member in hospital during treatment. This strong sense of family duty, and the resulting obligations, are amplified when accompanied by strong loyalty. It is important that this deep sense of duty is recognised and accommodated where possible.

The impact of spiritual beliefs on medical decision-making

This section provides a very brief overview of some of the cultural and spiritual groups nurses may encounter in clinical contexts. We may be describing your own cultural or religious group, or groups with which you may not be familiar. As a result, the descriptions are very brief and intended only as introductions.

In this way, you can build on your understanding of different groups as you progress through your study and clinical experiences. The list of cultures is also incomplete; there are many more religious and cultural groups that are not discussed here. What is important is the recognition that your patients' religious and cultural practices may not be either familiar to you or similar to your own views, so it is wise to respectfully ask about diet, holy days or other specific requirements for the followers of all spiritual and cultural beliefs during the provision of their care. Again, the practices outlined in Chapter 3 constitute appropriate ways to build your capacity for cross-cultural awareness and engagement.

Aboriginal and Torres Strait Islander peoples

There are a number of areas to consider when caring for an Aboriginal or Torres Strait Islander person. In Australia, the long negative history between non-Indigenous and Indigenous Australians since colonisation has resulted in understandable mistrust of broader community institutions, including hospitals, other healthcare environments and non-Indigenous healthcare providers. It is not possible in this short chapter to do justice to the complexities of the provision of Indigenous health. Clarke, Andrews and Austin (n.d.) recommend being mindful of cultural diversity, receptive and open, and demonstrating an understanding of Indigenous people and their needs in providing culturally safe care. The increasing numbers of Indigenous community healthcare services and Indigenous healthcare providers continue to improve cultural safety and provide non-Indigenous health professionals with valuable resources to develop healthcare for Indigenous people. There are a number of communication nuances that can impact effective communication. For many Indigenous people, direct eye contact with anyone other than close family and friends can be seen as rude, disrespectful or aggressive; therefore, in conversations, many Indigenous people tend to look down (Queensland Government, n.d.). So that Aboriginal and Torres Strait Islander peoples don't feel uncomfortable, you should sit beside them at a respectful distance in order to talk with them. Developing an understanding of complex kinship relationships, respect for community elders, strong connection with country and many other aspects of Aboriginal and Torres Strait Islander culture can assist in being able to provide culturally sensitive care. End-of-life care can also be complex, and 'sorry business'/'sad news' protocols associated with the death of a community member need to be respected. It is generally viewed as a point of respect not to display a photo of a deceased person, and this protocol may also extend to not speaking their name. Respect and recognition of gender segregation and 'men's business' and 'women's business' can be assisted by a same-sex care provider.

Buddhism

Followers of Buddhism are typically strictly vegetarian, and consideration of the non-use of any animal products in care or medicines is very important. The Buddhist concept of *samsara* (the cycle of life and rebirth), impermanence and the consequences of past-life experience (*karma*) can mean that people who follow a Buddhist tradition are accepting of various health conditions. The avoidance of intoxicants as part of the Buddhist faith may impact on a patient's acceptance of pain relief. In end-of-life care, underlying Buddhist beliefs can be a time of serious contemplation about their lived life and future life (reincarnation). Buddhist patients may request Buddhist clergy to assist them during their healthcare (Metropolitan Chicago Healthcare Council, 2005).

Christianity

All Christian religions are based on the teachings of the Christian Bible. There are many sub-groups of the Christian faith with specific needs: Roman Catholic, Anglican, Baptist, Lutheran, Methodist, Amish, Pentecostal, Church of Christ, Jehovah's Witness and many others. Some Christian groups have specific dietary requirements, including vegetarianism, or specific end-of-life requirements. People who follow Roman Catholicism are likely to observe Lent in the six weeks leading up to Easter, which may include special dietary requirements such as fasting or avoidance of meat. It is wise to ask about particular dietary or religious requirements on particular Christian holy days.

Hinduism

There are many aspects of Hinduism that will affect the way care is provided for a Hindu patient. Modesty is an important issue in both sexes, and a healthcare provider of one's own sex is preferred. Many Hindus wear a sacred thread or beads around the neck, waist or wrist, and permission should be sought before removing these items. Many follow a strict vegetarian diet;

those who eat meat do not eat beef or pork, and many have periods of fasting as part of their religious observance. It is also important to check medications to ensure they are not of animal origin, and a synthetic alternative should be offered where possible. There are many holy days, with particular observances for those days. The strong commitment to family may mean family members may request to stay overnight. There are many rituals associated with end-of-life care, including family members washing the body of the deceased family member, and having religious rituals conducted by a Pandit (priest), who may tie sacred threads or beads, or place other religious objects with the deceased person. These should not be removed without family permission.

Islam

People who follow Islam are known as Muslims, and have a number of specific religious requirements, including prayer, diet, washing and end-of-life care. Same-sex healthcare providers ensure strict modesty requirements for both sexes. It is important to ensure that women are kept covered, with only the face, hands and feet exposed. Men are similarly modest, with the area between the navel and knees strictly covered. The requirement for prayer on a special prayer mat five times each day should be accommodated; this is performed facing Mecca (the holy city of Islam). There are also important cleansing rituals associated with and performed before prayer. Muslims follow a strict *halal* diet, which excludes alcohol, pork products and any meat that has not been killed according to Islamic ritual. Food and medicines should be checked to ensure that they do not contain prohibited materials. Following the death of a relative, family members may request that the body face Mecca. Washing and shrouding the body should only be performed by family members according to Islamic requirements (Queensland Government, 2007b).

Judaism

Followers of Judaism adhere to the Old Testament scriptures known as the Torah. The holy day of Shabbat is observed from Friday to Saturday evening, and it is wise to ask about any kosher dietary or particular religious observances on holy days. Like all other religions, there are specific end-of-life requirements, and it is wise to respectfully ask.

Sikhism

There are particular dress rules associated with Sikhism, including wearing undergarments (men and woman) called *kachera* that should not be removed without permission. Similar sensitivity is required if there is a need to remove a man's turban (headdress) or women's scarves covering their hair, and these items should be treated with respect and never placed on the floor. There are many holy days on which particular rituals need to be observed, which may impact on medical treatment. Similarly, there are specific dietary requirements, which may impact on the type of medication someone is able to take. Many Sikhs follow a strict vegetarian diet, but those who do eat meat do not eat pork or beef, and only consume animals that have been killed by ritual slaughter (Queensland Government, 2007b). Death is generally accepted as a natural part of life, and specific religious needs should be discussed with individual patients.

Refugee patients

Another very diverse group of people you may meet in a clinical context are refugee patients. Several thousand people who have fled from their own unsafe countries and who are often affected by torture and trauma arrive in Australia as refugees every year. They often arrive with chronic, unmet physical and mental health challenges – particularly those who have experienced torture and trauma. For healthcare professionals, the particular needs of refugees are complex. Language barriers, cultural background, long periods of living in refugee camps and many other factors can contribute to poor physical and mental health, and this requires sensitive care that extends well beyond any cultural communication barriers. Refugees may experience poor concentration, insomnia, panic attacks, post-traumatic stress, depression, aggression and numerous other psychological and physical health problems, including chronic pain conditions. As a result of the trauma they have experienced, many refugees have problems with developing trust. Healthcare professionals need to be mindful of this in the provision of their care. Obtaining consent, taking time to explain various procedures and the reasons why they are required, and explaining medical equipment are crucial in the provision of all care (Queensland Government, 2013). In addition to these health problems, it is wise to gather information about the cultural background of the patient and any other particular dietary and healthcare requirements.

There will be many opportunities to meet students from different cultures and religions when you are studying or in a clinical context. Take advantage of these opportunities to increase your cross-cultural awareness by finding out more about these cultures and religions. Also take the opportunity to reflect on your developing understandings and apply this knowledge to your healthcare practices.

LEARNING ACTIVITY

Developing cross-cultural practices

The models of transition practices that help us identify the languages and practices in a new culture or context were introduced in Chapter 3. Here they are applied to an unfamiliar healthcare culture (see Figure 5.1).

If we can identify the key languages and literacies in the healthcare culture or context we are entering as students on clinical placements or as registered nurses, we will be better equipped to make a comfortable transition to a new culture. An essential part of this process is our examination of and reflection on our own cultural self-awareness, cultural values, attitudes, beliefs and practices. This is

Financial management
Administrative practices
Human resource practices
Shift practices
Employment practices
Social practices
Codes of conduct and ethics
Patients' cultures

Healthcare context

Union requirements
Stress management
Time management
Computer technology
Ward and clinical practices
Hospital practices
Organisational culture
Balancing work and home life

FIGURE
5.1
Languages and practices in a healthcare context

to ensure that we are able to overcome any cultural stereotypes that may impact on the provision of judgement-free healthcare. In the competency standards for nurses, the Australian Nursing and Midwifery Council (2008) notes that nurses not only need to respect the diversity of beliefs of colleagues and those in their care, but develop competence in accommodating those beliefs.

 When you are on your next clinical placement, identify the cultures, religions, languages and practices present. Reflect on what you can do to become familiar with, understand and develop your knowledge about these cultures and practices.

Reflective practice

Reflective practice includes developing your awareness of, respect for and patience with the practices and languages in the new context. Listening and observation are central to engaging with the new context and its languages and literacies. It is also important to act appropriately and respectfully; in this way, you will be aware of and demonstrate your professionalism.

 After identifying the new languages and practices you need to become familiar with and demonstrate on your next clinical placement, reflect on the best ways to demonstrate your respect for these practices:
> What is your clinical uniform and how do you wear it? What are the most appropriate shoes to wear?
> What are the shift changeover practices?
> Are there forms you need to complete?
> Are there different cultures present in the workplace, and do you need to adjust your thinking to accommodate these groups' practices?

Communication practice

Communication practice is your capacity to seek help, make social contact and participate in a group. These practices also work in reverse. For example, you could be the expert issuing advice and support, or you could be a nurse helping a new patient or new staff member to become familiar by using your communication practices. You could use common words: be aware of your own use of slang and colloquial expressions and avoid using them; be alert to being misunderstood and ask if your message was clear; watch for non-verbal signals (facial expressions) that can alert you to any misunderstandings, and seek to clarify; and paraphrase important points.

Case study

This is an email that I received from one of the staff members working with refugee students, describing some of the difficulties they experienced in using appropriate and expected communication practices in the Australian higher education culture.

> Refugees come from countries with no tradition or custom of seeking assistance from authorities (who may be downright dangerous to approach) or any concept of our counsellors. This, along with communication issues, makes it very difficult to enter the established complaints system if they have concerns about academic issues or relationship issues that may impact on study: for example, problems with group work, not getting fair treatment from a staff member, etc. This is especially an issue on nursing clinical where they may have problems with hospital staff and are unwilling or unable to express themselves to academic staff back at the university over issues that are affecting their work.
>
> This is a very serious matter as I have experienced a number of first-year students who give up and leave because of issues I think an Australian student would have been more likely to resolve by seeking help from student support services or the student ombudsmen.
>
> Also I have experienced a number of occasions when student services staff have not understood the student or not persevered with helping them to resolve their issues. Students often resist even going to seek help.

Critical reflection

What are the communication practices you can use to fine-tune the skills and strategies you need to exhibit to receive a positive outcome for clinical? Think about:

〉〉 Who are the people in practice to whom you have found yourself looking for advice? How did you approach them?

〉〉 Are there groups or work-based classes you could join, such as morning tea groups?

Critical practice

As outlined in Chapter 3, critical practice involves both an awareness of your belief systems and cultural practices, and an awareness of the power relationships in operation around you. Critical practice also involves the ability to seek and give feedback about specific higher education practices and belief systems. The previous case study is actually an example of the power relationships that sometimes operate between students and staff in both academic and clinical contexts.

What are the critical practices you can fine-tune to receive a positive outcome for your clinical experience? Think about the following:

> What were your expectations about the clinical context in which you were practising, and how did these differ from the reality?

> What behaviours or communication practices did you notice that surprised you?

> What taken-for-granted assumptions did you have about the staff and patients at clinical?

> Did you observe any occasions where staff needed to provide you with feedback about your performance? What strategies did they use? Were these effective?

As in the previous discussion about communication practice, the situation could occur in reverse: you could be the expert. You can use the same critical practices to assist others to move comfortably into your culture or context. For example, you could clarify any situation by asking for feedback: 'Are you comfortable when …?'; Can you explain to me how …?'; 'Was it clear to you when I said …?'; 'Tell me how often you are going to take your medication.'

Dynamic practices

As Chapter 3 suggested, these practices are dynamic – they overlap and intersect with each other. For example, asking for help may intersect with the skill of requesting feedback. Both these skills and practices are combined when using an interpreter to communicate with patients – when obtaining consent, taking the time to explain various procedures and the reasons they are required, or explaining the use of medical equipment.

Tips for working with interpreters

The services of an accredited interpreter should always be used during all conversations about care, when consent is required (for instance, for surgery), about medication, at admission and discharge, and at other times where this is considered necessary by the lack of ability of the person to understand your verbal or written communication due to language differences. Accredited interpreters should always be used except in a medical emergency, where no accredited interpreter is available.

- Never use a person younger than 18 years of age as an interpreter.
- Allow adequate time (about twice as long as a regular interview of the same type).

- If the interpreter is in the same room, sit in a triangular formation.
- If the interpreter is interpreting by phone, ensure you have a speakerphone or a dual-handset phone.
- Ensure the interpreter understands that they are bound by a strict code of ethics regarding confidentiality.
- Ensure the patient feels safe and understands what the discussion is about.
- Look directly at the patient being interviewed, and stop to allow the interpreter to interpret after two to three sentences.
- Address the patient – for example, 'How is your wound healing?'
- Ask one question at a time.
- Avoid the use of medical terms and colloquial expressions.
- Make use of diagrams and written material in the patient's language if available.
- Regularly summarise the conversation.
- Be specific, particularly when summarising discharge care – for example, 'Take medication X at six in the morning, at midday and at six in the evening', not 'Take medication X regularly'.
- Clarify that you have been understood and encourage questions from the patient.
- Debrief the interpreter after the interview if the conversation is difficult (Queensland Government, 2007a).

Summary

Once we understand that we are part of a culture and a member of a number of cultural groups, we may need to shift some of the understandings we have about the world. We can no longer accept there is just one 'right' way of knowing and behaving. There may be other ways that are just as appropriate in other cultures and cultural groups. To be effective communicators, we need to recognise that uncertainty may arise when we communicate because we may be crossing others' ways of knowing, and their world-views and perceptions.

Cultural sensitivity involves using a number of practices. We need to reflect on who we are, and about the beliefs, values, expectations, skills and knowledge we have developed as members of a range of cultural groups. We also need to be able to explore both our negative and positive responses to cultural difference or diversity. For example, we need to investigate whether our negative responses may have emerged from the expectations, assumptions and stereotypes we hold about others' ways of understanding the world. We also need to build on our more positive responses to develop cultural competence or literacy, and to understand that adapting to diversity and communicating across cultures is a process of lifelong learning.

Cultural sensitivity also involves reflecting about the practices, languages and literacies present in both our own culture and unfamiliar cultures with which we are engaging. As experts in our own culture, we can help make our cultural practices clear and explicit to newcomers to our culture. As newcomers to another culture, we can use practices like asking for help, making social contact and participating in groups to become more effective in engaging the literacies and languages of the new culture.

Cultural sensitivity also involves our awareness of our own belief systems and cultural practices (critical self-awareness) as well as an awareness of the power relationships in operation around us.

Building our capacities to exhibit cultural sensitivity evolves as we grow personally, as we travel and as we develop relationships with people who differ from us. The good news is that moving beyond the belief that ours is the only 'right' way shifts us to a place that allows us to understand and respect difference, and to communicate across cultures, transforming ourselves in the process.

The strength of the practices is that they move beyond cultural binaries by placing each of us (regardless of the context or culture being engaged) on an intercultural journey. The practices instil in us a resilience that enables us to apply and reapply these practices so we are empowered to meet each new challenge as it emerges in the fast-moving and complex world in which we live. The practices help us understand what is cultural about our own and others' understandings, including those of the higher education and the health-care world, and how to apply these understandings in their engagement with other groups and cultures. Together, the practices illustrate a form of 'lifelong learning'.

Discussion and critical thinking questions

5.1 Think about a culture or cultural group with which you are familiar and identify the cultural practices, literacies and languages present in the culture.

5.2 Explain why you think it is important to develop your intercultural or transcultural skills.

5.3 What strategies will you use to engage with an unfamiliar cultural context?

5.4 How can you apply these skills so they become lifelong learning skills, which will empower you to cope with the continual change in contemporary healthcare?

Learning extension

Think of the clinical environments in which you have worked.

- What are the similarities and differences between these contexts?
- How many cultural groups exist in the same clinical environment?
- Do they communicate in the same ways?
- Are some groups more productive and focused than others in their reflective, communication and critical practices? Does this disparity have something to do with their cultural behaviours and practices?
- If you had the chance to go back to one or other of these clinical areas, what ideas might you have for doing things differently? How is this approach linked to the actions of a clinical leader?

Further reading

Hazelwood, Z. & Shakespeare-Finch, J. (2010). *Let's talk: Communication for health professionals*. Sydney: Pearson Australia.

References

Andrews, M.M. & Boyle, J.S. (2002). Transcultural concepts in nursing care. *Journal of Transcultural Nursing*, 13(3): 178–80.

Australian Bureau of Statistics (ABS) (2013). *Australian social trends: Doctors and nurses*. Canberra: ABS. Retrieved 10 July 2014 from <http://www.abs.gov.au/ausstats/abs@.nsf/Lookup/4102.0Main±Features 20April±2013#p7>.

Australian Commission on Safety and Quality in Health Care (ACSQHC) (2006). *National terminology, abbreviations and symbols to be used in the prescribing and administering of medicines in Australian hospitals*. Canberra: ACSQHC. Retrieved 5 July 2014 from <http://www.health.wa.gov.au/CircularsNew/attachments/383.pdf>.

Australian Health Practitioner Regulation Agency (AHPRA) (2014). *Registration requirements*. Retrieved 5 July 2014 from <http://www.ahpra.gov.au/Registration/RegistrationProcess/Registration-Requirements.aspx>.

Australian Nursing and Midwifery Council (ANMC) (2008). *Code of professional conduct for nurses in Australia*. Canberra: ANMC.

Clarke, A., Andrews, S. & Austin, N. (n.d). *Lookin' after our own: Supporting Aboriginal families through the hospital experience*. Melbourne: Aboriginal Family Support Unit – Royal Children's Hospital.

Hazelwood, Z. & Shakespeare-Finch, J. (2010). *Let's talk: Communication for health professionals*. Sydney: Pearson Australia.

Hofstede, G. (2001). *Culture's consequences: Comparing values, behaviors, institutions, and organizations across nations*. Thousand Oaks, CA: Sage.

—— (2014). *Gerte Hofstede: Culture*. Retrieved 4 July 2014 from <http://geerthofstede.nl/culture>.

Kossen, C., Kiernan, E. & Lawrence, J. (eds) (2013). *Communicating for success*. Sydney: Pearson Australia.

Kuokkanen, L. & Leino-Kilpi, H. (2000). Power and empowerment in nursing: Three theoretical approaches. *Journal of Advanced Nursing*, 31(1): 235–41.

Lankshear, C., Gee, P., Knobel, M. & Searle, C. (1997). *Changing literacies*. Maidenhead: Open University Press.

Lawrence, J. (2014). Living comfortably with diversity: International students' transition practices. *Queensland Review*, 21(2): 217–32.

McGarty, C., Yzerbyt, V.Y. & Spears, R. (2002). Social, cultural and cognitive factors in stereotype formation. In C. McGarty (ed.), *Stereotypes as explanations: The formation of meaningful beliefs about social groups*. Melbourne: Cambridge University Press, pp. 1–15.

Metropolitan Chicago Healthcare Council (MCHC) (2005). *Quick reference for health care providers interacting with Buddhist patients and their families*. Chicago: MCHC. Retrieved 20 January 2015 from <http://info.kyha.com/documents/QR-ALL.pdf>.

Queensland Government (2007a). *Working with interpreters: Guidelines*. Brisbane: Queensland Health.

—— (2007b). *Cultural profiles*. Brisbane: Queensland Health. Retrieved 5 July 2014 from <http://www.health.qld.gov.au/multicultural/health_workers/cultdiver_guide.asp>.

—— (2013). *Torture and trauma: A guide for health professionals*. Brisbane: Queensland Health.

—— (n.d.). *Communicating effectively with Aboriginal and Torres Strait Islander people*. Brisbane: Queensland Health. Retrieved 20 January 2015 from <http://www.health.qld.gov.au/deadly_ears/docs/hp-res-comeffect.pdf>.

Scott, G., Ciarrochi, J. & Deane, F.P. (2004). Disadvantages of being an individualist in an individualistic culture: Idiocentrism, emotional competence, stress, and mental health. *Australian Psychologist*, 39(2): 143–54.

Suominen, T., Krovatin, M. & Ketola, O. (1997). Nursing culture: Some viewpoints. *Journal of Advanced Nursing*, 25: 186–90.

Developing interpersonal capabilities for healthcare professionals

6

Julie Martyn and Eleanor Kiernan

Learning objectives

- Identify why effective communication is important and how professional standards can contribute to effective communication in healthcare settings.

- Understand how nurses' self-concept can influence the effectiveness of their communication.

- Recognise that non-verbal communication is central to nursing care and that it is multidimensional.

- Understand the significance of bullying in nursing practice.

- Evaluate strategies that address bullying.

Key terms

- Chronemics

- Haptics

- Kinesics

- Oculesics

- Paralinguistics

- Self-awareness

- Self-concept

- Self-efficacy

- Workplace bullying

Introduction

Effective communication is crucial in many professions, but it is particularly important in the nursing profession. Nurses who are poor communicators can make a patient's stay in hospital unhappy or uncomfortable, and in extreme cases poor communication could have life or death implications. For these reasons, it is imperative that nurses have an understanding of the importance of possessing strong communication skills and that they are capable of exhibiting them in healthcare settings and beyond. This chapter considers nursing's professional standards in global and local contexts to show how central effective communication is to nursing practice. The chapter also builds on understandings about how a nurse's communication skills can be improved by honest self-evaluation achieved by reflection. The practice of reflection can promote **self-awareness** that facilitates effective change, resulting in improved communication skills. Advanced communication skills help nurses to meet the interpersonal challenges they encounter, such as bullying. The impact of bullying on the individual and the organisation is explored along with strategies to minimise and manage such destructive behaviour. These strategies are evaluated at the end of the chapter.

> **self-awareness:** an individual's insight into their own behaviour; acknowledging personal strengths and weaknesses

Nursing standards in global and local contexts

Care providers' communication capabilities are valued from international and national perspectives. Across the globe, nursing's scope of practice incorporates the competencies and accountabilities of the nurse's capacity to respond to change (ICN, 2013). Individually, a nurse's scope of practice is not limited to tasks, functions or responsibilities, but rather relies on a combination of knowledge, judgement and skills (ICN, 2013). Nurses' responsibilities include coordinating the inputs of the interdisciplinary healthcare team members to determine a comprehensive plan for patient care (Dempsey, Hillege & Hill, 2014). The range of responsibilities means the nurse needs to be a versatile and emotionally intelligent communicator.

Various international health organisations, both globally and locally, emphasise the importance of teamwork in their policies as an important ingredient of patient safety. For example, the World Health Organization (WHO) has a mandate to strengthen the capacity of the nursing and midwifery workforce through strategies to forge strong interdisciplinary health teams (WHO, 2014). This includes being able to function effectively in a healthcare team made up of professionals from multiple disciplines. The International Council of Nurses (ICN, 2013) recognises that nursing is known to be allied to other professions through collaborating, referring and coordinating healthcare activities.

In Australia, the national competency standards for registered nurses work in conjunction with the Nursing and Midwifery Board of Australia (NMBA) registration standards, and are used as the criteria to determine a person's right to be registered or enrolled as a practising nurse (NMBA, 2014). Australian nursing standards are broad, and cover professional issues related to continuing professional development, criminal history disclosure, English language skills, professional indemnity arrangements, recency of practice, various endorsements and eligibilities (NMBA, 2014). The competencies are more specific to an individual's professional practice, and their capability and capacity to demonstrate, under the domains of professional practice, critical thinking and analysis, provision and coordination of care and collaboration and therapeutic practice (NMBA, 2006).

Communication is a core ability mentioned in each of these competency domains in terms of the nurse demonstrating skills in protecting human rights, and appraisal of and feedback about self and others through reflective practice. Coordination and delegation of care with and for others, and establishing successful therapeutic and professional relationships, are also core competencies (NMBA, 2006). Competency standards in New Zealand also include specific indicators related to establishing rapport and relationships based on trust, respect and empathy (Nursing Council of New Zealand, 2014).

Beyond the professional requirements of nursing is the need to understand how nurses' behaviours and communication styles affect their patients' perceptions of their healthcare experience. As nurses are ever-present in the healthcare setting, it is their responsibility to consistently provide physical, psychological and emotional support to people receiving healthcare services. This recognition is coupled with the knowledge that effective interpersonal communication is crucial if nurses are to respond to changes in the contexts of contemporary healthcare while balancing the often competing demands of advancing work practices and complex client needs (Glass, 2010).

Interpersonal communication in healthcare settings

Interpersonal communication is at the heart of nursing. It can be defined as a 'cyclic, reciprocal, interactive, and dynamic process, with value, cultural, and cognitive variables that influence its transmission and reception' (Arnold & Underman Boggs, 2011, p. 13). Nurses encounter numerous communication challenges in their work. The consequence of this is that in a typical shift nurses interact with patients about a variety of issues concerning their health. For example, nurses collaborate and negotiate with other healthcare providers; they manage and lead members of the healthcare team; and they delegate and instruct health service staff. Nurses therefore need the mental agility to cope with and respond to the bombardment of messages they receive over the course of a shift. Logical and critical thinking is also required to prioritise the messages so that appropriate clinical decisions can be made. Advanced verbal, non-verbal and written communications techniques are then needed to disseminate and communicate the decisions reached. Nurses develop these communication and critical thinking skills throughout their careers, but their awareness of the need to develop such skills is established as early as their first year of study as nursing students.

The understanding of the extent and complexity of the communication, as well as the type and frequency of interpersonal communication that occurs for nurses, is reflected in some research studies – for example, in a UK emergency department, researchers measured the number of communication events with which a head nurse had to deal in a shift. They found that the head nurse had over 1000 separate communication events over a 10-hour shift (Woloshynowych et al., 2007). This seems an extraordinary number, but they uncovered even more sobering facts: 14 per cent of these communication situations were simultaneous and 30 per cent were interruptions to a task. This research illustrates that nurses have to mentally juggle a host of competing pressures in an emergency department, where attention needs to be focused on urgent emergency situations. In stressful circumstances where expectations are high and there are many demands, nurses need both robust and dynamic communication skills to negotiate these demands successfully. To achieve this, they need to learn the skills and be prepared to practise them as they progress through their degree and clinical placement experience.

Nurses encounter and engage with many different people in the course of their day. They also need to prioritise the messages as they receive them – which can be challenging, because they are subject to competing demands. For example, a patient may need analgesia, a doctor may be demanding assistance, a ward clerk needs bed availability and the hospitality staff want to know where to take a patient's meal. Conflict arises if the clinical decisions or priorities of the nurse are impacted by these differing needs. Some of these stresses can sometimes erupt into aggressive behaviour – indeed, aggression and violence in the emergency department are common. Nurses are exposed to it more than other healthcare and emergency services workers (Hodge & Marshall, 2007), as patients presenting to emergency departments have expectations that their injury or illness will be reviewed and managed quickly.

Building self-awareness and self-concept

Previous chapters have identified how personal beliefs and biases influence the way we think and communicate with others. It is important for nurses to gain insight and to understand the personal perceptions and prejudices that might affect the therapeutic relationships they are expected to establish with patients. Self-awareness and experience contribute to the development of effective communication skills. Stein-Parbury (2014) suggests, for example, that if nurses are authentic, sincere and genuine with patients, they will develop a more open and meaningful relationship with them.

Think back to a recent incident where you were involved in a disagreement. On reflection, do you now think you were in the wrong? If so, what has helped to develop your self-awareness to the extent that you can now look at the situation more objectively? Will this have an impact on the way you interact with the other person in the future? Write a paragraph about the insights you have developed about your increasing self-awareness.

A level of self-awareness is integral to identifying weaknesses, building strengths and overcoming 'blind spots' – for example, in coordinating patient care in clinical contexts. Blind spots are those places where communication gaps occur that are potentially harmful to patients, and to organisational objectives and outcomes. The Johari window (created by Luft and Ingham in the 1950s and still relevant today) is a self-awareness model created as four quadrants displaying aspects of levels of self-awareness. The quadrants are: *known to self, known to others, hidden* and *unknown to self.* The Johari window (see Luft, 1984) outlines the progressive nature of self-awareness from unknown to open. The two quadrants that are important to the discussion in this chapter are the *known to self* and *unknown to self* (or blind) quadrants. The more self-aware we become, the fewer blind spots we have, and if we act on this knowledge we can improve our interpersonal communication.

To transition from the blind spot to a place where personal characteristics are known to self and others requires a deep understanding of the self. Nurses who already have a realistic understanding of themselves have a useful starting point in their communication and behaviour. For example, if a busy shift consistently makes a nurse short-tempered, but there is self-realisation about this, then there is a strong basis for change. Insight can provide nurses with information from which to enhance or halt specific ways of behaving. Conversely, nurses who are oblivious that their behaviour is negatively affecting colleagues and patients will be hampered in terms of improving the situation.

It can be difficult for most people to alter long-standing behaviours, but in circumstances where there is limited insight, it is very difficult and might require feedback from others to inspire a change. Behavioural change is dependent upon the inspiration and motivation of the individual. Motivation contributes to and is a key attribute of self-awareness (Dempsey, Hillege & Hill, 2014). The nursing competency standards are strong external motivators for seeking to gain personal insight and being alert to improvement opportunities. The care and safety of the patient are also powerful external motivators. Internal motivation is required when attempting to improve interpersonal capabilities in nursing practice, and this can be the most challenging thing of all. For example, the nurse may feel strongly motivated purely to improve the level of care they give to the patient.

Reflective practice

Self-awareness is a component of reflective practice, which is central to changing behaviour for improving nursing practice. As Chapter 3 outlined, reflection involves thinking about one's nursing practice and communication, and how these affect others or can be improved. There are certain conditions that help reflective skills to flourish. These conditions, according to Mann, Gordon and McLeod (2009, cited in Devenny & Duffy, 2013, p. 38) include:

- intellectual and emotional support
- an authentic context (that is, within an organisational climate that promotes respect between professionals)
- access to mentoring

- time for group discussion and reflection
- freedom of expression of opinions.

Reflective practice is made up of purposeful actions and exercises, and is a creative process. Glass (2010) offers a model for reflecting on self to increase personal awareness. This includes listening to the substance of the messages you communicate to yourself. Sometimes, the substance of what we say to ourselves can be positive and at other times can be negative and detrimental to the **self-concept**. For example, if a nursing student were treated badly by a patient, the student could look at it in a negative light which could damage the student's self-concept; however, if the student chose to look at it as a learning opportunity rather than a personal failure, then the self-concept could actually be enhanced. This approach reflects Glass's (2010) recommendation about reframing such troublesome or counterproductive self-talk into positive responses. Improving one's self-perception in this way will promote self-efficacy (see below) through an enriched self-concept.

self-concept:
the way we view ourselves; self-concept is not necessarily accurate

Imagine you are enrolled in a course of study. This course has a quiz as the final piece of assessment. To pass the course, you must pass the quiz. But when the results of the quiz are returned, you received 45/100.

> Examine your inner dialogue right now.
> Is what you are saying to yourself nurturing or negative?

Your response to the learning activity is most likely negative, and may sound something like, 'This is terrible. I failed. I should have studied more.' Negative self-talk is harmful rather than helpful. Alternatively, more realistic and positive dialogue might include, 'This result is not what I hoped for. Does the course offer supplementary work? It means I may have to do the course again. I need to make an appointment with the examiner to discuss my options. If necessary, another attempt at the course will help me to get better grades next time.'

Self-efficacy and assertiveness

Self-efficacy is a valuable attribute that contributes to effective communication. People who practise self-efficacy recognise and value their strengths and abilities, and can motivate themselves towards meeting challenges by regulating their thoughts and feelings (Moyle, Parker & Bramble, 2014). Self-awareness is therefore strongly associated with self-efficacy (Arnold & Underman Boggs, 2011). As noted

self-efficacy:
self-belief in a person's strengths and abilities to achieve their goals

previously, reflection is a way by which nurses can improve their competency in these and other aspects of their practice.

Assertiveness is an important skill because it is based on respect for self and others. It does not reflect a 'win at all costs' mentality, but rather respects and accounts for the rights of individuals. An assertive nurse or nursing student can use skills to try to resolve the problem. If there is a dispute between healthcare practitioners, the assertive skills of the nurse will be useful. Respecting your rights and those of others sounds counter-intuitive when you are in a dispute; however, you need to be aware that the other person may have a different perspective and that you need to negotiate a common understanding. The key to assertiveness is to take the emotion out of the situation, as emotion usually exacerbates the problem. The person needs to calmly state the problem, articulate its impact and try to look at the problem from the other person's point of view. A solution should then be offered. (Chapters 2 and 3 include some of the practical strategies for being assertive.) Some of the hallmarks of assertiveness include being able to provide constructive feedback, having the confidence to ask for feedback and being able to say 'no' without feeling guilty. This is an important tool in the nursing context – particularly when there are competing demands from colleagues and patients.

Non-verbal communication

Types of non-verbal communication

The nurse's non-verbal communication has a powerful and important impact on the delivery of care. Non-verbal communication can be defined as communication without words, but this simple definition belies its complexity. Non-verbal communication is more than body language; it incorporates many different elements, some of which are:

- **kinesics** (body language), including movement, gestures, facial expressions and gesticulations)
- **oculesics** – linked to kinesics, this refers to the study of eye behaviour
- **haptics** – communication through touch
- **chronemics** – relates to use and perception of time
- **paralinguistics** – the tone of our voice.

kinesics:
non-verbal behaviour relating to body movement (facial expressions, gestures, gesticulations and movement); body language

oculesics:
non-verbal communication relating to eye behaviour

haptics:
non-verbal communication relating to touch

chronemics:
non-verbal communication relating to how time is interpreted

paralinguistics:
the tone of voice that can convey a non-verbal message

An understanding of the different types of non-verbal communication can help nurses to identify and consider where adjustments might be made to positively contribute to patient care. The non-verbal communication methods applicable to the nursing context are discussed below.

Kinesics and oculesics are two types of non-verbal communication that are closely linked. A nurse's alertness to these non-verbal messages can help to progress the nurse–patient dialogue so that common understanding is achieved. The patient may say one thing but the non-verbal cues could undermine the spoken message.

Kinesics is body language. It denotes how we move, what gestures and gesticulations we use, our deportment and the way we walk. Our body language can betray our words at times. For example, on inquiring about a patient's health, an answer of 'Fine, thank you' could be accompanied by slouched shoulders and a downward gaze. The body language here is contradicting the spoken language. Even people who are aware of the impact of body language and try to 'match' their spoken and non-verbal aspects by smiling and appearing cheerful will be exposed by incongruent or conflicting cues. A nurse who is aware that monitoring for this incongruence can provide valuable information for guiding necessary patient care will respond and question the patient further.

Oculesics relates to how people use their eyes, and can be a way to regulate and progress the communication as well as closing the psychological distance between people. Eye contact can also stall communication – particularly when there are variables such as culture, gender, age and status inhibiting its effectiveness. In Australia, eye contact is regarded as a measure of a person's confidence and honesty. However, some cultures avoid eye contact as a sign of respect to the status of the person. If the nurse is unaware of this, it can be misinterpreted and complicate care. This is where the negotiation of meaning is so important (see Chapter 2 and Chapter 5). The nurse can clarify confusions or concerns respectfully if this occurs.

Gaze and eye contact between the nurse and patient can be a key source of information and comfort. There are some patients who cannot speak because of conditions such as stroke, who rely on non-verbal communication to try to convey their feelings. Their eyes may be the only channel of communication. By paying special attention to the eyes of a patient during all interactions, the nurse has the opportunity to collect information that can contribute to comprehensive care. For example, squinting might indicate pain or discomfort, so further investigation at this point is warranted.

Coupled with verbal messages such as greeting by name and use of gesture, eye contact is recognised as a positive communication behaviour. A lack of eye contact by the nurse is a significant variable determining how successful the communication exchange is perceived to be by the patient (Happ et al., 2011). Nurses therefore need to be aware of the importance of using the eyes to gauge information and to help allay anxiety. However, cultural differences can affect the interpretation of eye contact, as in some cultures eye contact is determined by status. Children, for example, are trained not to look directly at their elders when speaking to them (Maier-Lorentz, 2008). These cultural differences may seem to be insurmountable, as there are so many variations. However, Maier-Lorentz (2008, p. 39) states that 'nurses must be cognizant that several meanings may be attached to direct eye contact in order to communicate effectively with their patients'. It is therefore worth building knowledge as both a nursing student and a nurse. And it is worth remembering that not all people conform to a cultural expectation, which further complicates the issue.

Haptics is a type of non-verbal communication that relates to touch, and is sometimes viewed with suspicion in professional contexts. For example, teachers often modify their initial response to comfort a distressed child by hugging the child because of concern about using inappropriate touch. The use of haptics by nurses, however, is generally not viewed suspiciously, as most people see it as necessary and therapeutic. Therapeutic touch can be a powerful tool when used at the right time (Hillege, Hardy & Glew, 2014). Nurses practise in the intimate space of patients, and providing care by gently touching the patient's hand or patting the shoulder can be encouraging and comforting for some. However, touch can also be quite confronting for the patient, even though they know it is necessary. Because healthcare practices involve nurses entering the personal and intimate space of others, there are inherent risks of patients becoming uncomfortable despite the sensitivity of the nurse (Glass, 2010). Therefore, the way a patient is touched by the nurse is extremely important and must be congruent with the intervention required. When used appropriately, touch is an effective form of communication; however, touching another person can have a multiplicity of interpretations for the receiver. Some factors that influence the way someone interprets the touch of another are family, religion, class, culture, age and gender (Hillege, Hardy & Glew, 2014, p. 119). Some cultures, for instance, have a more tactile and less inhibited approach while others have strong values and beliefs that prohibit, for example, male nurses touching females. It doesn't necessarily have to be intimate touch, as in some Asian countries touching of the head is not welcomed because the head is seen to be the source of a person's strength (Maier-Lorentz, 2008). If nursing students learn about such cultural differences during their studies, they will become sensitised to these differences and try to be culturally sensitive where possible (see Chapter 5).

Chronemics is a dimension of non-verbal communication that is different from the types discussed above because it doesn't relate to one-on-one interaction with the various cues given and interpreted. Chronemics relates to time – that is, a message is conveyed about a person by their use of time. For example, a university student who arrives late to class every week may be judged as being uninterested, rude or even lazy. The fact that the student may not be able to get there because of a clash of class times or bus schedules is not considered by the observers. This kind of misunderstanding can be present in healthcare. How we use our time sends a message to others that can contain value judgements. In the nursing context, the amount of time spent with a patient may not be as much as the patient would hope. The patient may interpret this as them being less valued by the nurse. However, the reality may be that resources are stretched and the nurse could be overwhelmed with work pressures. It is disappointing that these stretched resources can affect the time spent with patients and their families, as these discussions could actually help to save time in the long run; time spent talking to patients and relatives can help nurses to recognise nuances in individual treatment responses (Chan, Jones & Wong, 2013, p. 2026). Nurses often need to have discussions about their capacity to deliver care. Openly communicating with the patient can help to avoid misunderstandings by establishing expectations. Nurses in the emergency department are frequently responding to inquiries about perceived delays in treatment from patients with non-urgent conditions. Talking to those involved about the realities of the nurse's time constraints can help to lower expectations and anxiety.

Paralinguistics (or vocalics) refers to the tone of the voice. It can reinforce the spoken message or it can undermine it. When an impatient or hostile tone is used, it has the potential to increase anxiety in a patient. The patient is already in a vulnerable position. 'It is important for healthcare providers to be aware of the power of voice tone and consider how their emotions may be inadvertently leaked through their voice tone.' (Haskard et al., 2008, p. 18). Healthcare is a complex and busy environment, and some non-verbal messages can be (unwittingly) detrimental to patient care (see Thomas's story on page 143). For example, if anger is conveyed to the patient, it could serve to weaken the trust that is so pivotal to the healthcare setting. Consider the nurse who disregards a patient's requests for analgesia because the nurse does not believe the patient requires the medication.

An understanding of the different types of non-verbal communication can help nurses to identify and consider where adjustments might be made to positively contribute to patient care.

The relationship between verbal and non-verbal communication

Nurses' awareness of their non-verbal messages may help to convey a sense of confidence, warmth and empathy to the patient, particularly when the non-verbal behaviour is positively linked to verbal communication. Problems emerge, however, when there is a lack of congruency between the verbal and non-verbal messages. For example, the nurse may use positive and encouraging words, but the message could be undermined by incongruent non-verbal messages such as hostile tone of voice or less than gentle handling of the patient. Much of our non-verbal behaviour is seemingly inherent, and it takes a concerted effort to change the way we use particular cues. Patients may exhibit stoic or bravado behaviours when in fact they may be deeply anxious about their circumstances. A nurse who is astute at detecting this by actively listening and observing can gather a great deal more information that could then generate new directions in patient–nurse conversations, which in turn could ultimately help guide patient care. For example, incongruence of facial expressions and body language with spoken responses is a sign for the nurse to ask more questions to gain greater insight.

Brad's Story

Case study

Critical reflection

Brad Smith is a 17-year-old male patient admitted to a surgical ward with acute appendicitis. He had laparoscopic surgery yesterday and is expected to be ambulant within a day. In preparation for mobilising him, the nurse offers him analgesia. Brad's response is, 'Nah, I'll be right. It's only a small wound.' He attempts to move in the bed, his eyes squint, his mouth grimaces and he guards his abdomen with his hands.

》 What are the non-verbal cues or signals that are incongruent with Brad's spoken words?

》 Why do you think Brad is trying to be stoic despite his obvious pain and discomfort?

Non-verbal communication makes up a significant part of a message, and can change how the message is received. A nurse who is unaware of the impact of non-verbal communication can miss opportunities in patient care. However, nurses can also positively contribute to patient care when they pay attention to non-verbal signals. For example, the nurse must take time to practise therapeutic presence by actively listening to the patient, observing their body language, considering their condition and investigating by questioning when the data gathered are inconsistent or concerning. Geller (2012) describes therapeutic presence as an intentional act of focusing fully on the interaction with the patient. By being fully engaged with the patient, the nurse is in the best position to get a clearer message from which to act on or enable patient-centred care.

Active or attentive listening is one way to demonstrate therapeutic presence. Attentive listening involves the nurse or nursing student taking the time to completely engage with what the patient is saying. To do this, distractions must be ignored unless there is an emergency. Reflecting understanding of the issue back to the patient and seeking clarity from them ensures that the message has been understood correctly. Nurses who listen attentively to patient experiences are able to collect concrete and personally unique data on which they can base patient-centred nursing interventions (Stein-Parbury, 2014). Brad's story illustrates how the patient's words may not reflect the reality of the situation.

Non-verbal communication can be misinterpreted

Non-verbal cues are important to gauge the full message; however, they are also very susceptible to misinterpretation, so the whole range of cues and the links between the verbal and non-verbal messages need to be considered. A perceptive nurse will identify the incongruent non-verbal and verbal messages and explore further, as in Brad's case. People can be sensitive to the slightest shift in non-verbal behaviour. Knowing a person's baseline behaviour (their normal pattern of behaviour) can help to pinpoint contradictions between the spoken word and the non-verbal behaviour or cues. This is particularly important in the nurse–patient relationship, as the non-verbal aspects can be vital – particularly if the patient is scared or too ill to speak, and is reliant on the nurse to try to understand what is happening. In intensive care units, patients are sometimes desperate to communicate, and may only have their eyes and their arms/legs to convey their level of pain (Happ et al., 2011). It is therefore important that the nurse looks for and tries to understand such non-verbal signals.

Thomas's story

Case study

I have been nursing for ten years at a busy metropolitan hospital and pride myself on my communication with my patients. I always try to be cheerful around them, as I think that will make their illness more manageable. This approach usually works, and patients are generally pleased to see me.

That's before I was assigned to care for Marie. I always greeted her in a light-hearted way. My tone of voice was sunny and I thought it was quite endearing. Other patients seemed to respond well to my approach. Marie was different. There seemed to be an invisible barrier between her and me. I tried patting her on the hand, laughing, telling jokes but it was all to no avail. She just didn't respond to me. I was surprisingly upset about it.

Eventually, I decided to ask her how we could improve our communication. I asked her if I'd done anything to offend her, as she seemed reluctant to talk to me. At first she said 'No, there's nothing wrong'. I persisted, however, and eventually she told me that she thought I was patronising, that the tone of my voice sounded like I was talking to a child.

I was flabbergasted and in denial! However, I reflected on her comments over the next couple of days and I realised she was right. I tried hard to use a more respectful tone, not just to Marie but to other patients. I still use humour and a light tone, but it is definitely less patronising. Marie responded well because she knew I had made a conscious effort to change based on her feedback.

Critical reflection

>> What type of non-verbal communication was Thomas addressing?

>> Why do you think some of the patients did not have a negative reaction to Thomas's style?

>> If you received constructive criticism about your communication style, how would you go about reflecting on your practice? What questions would you ask yourself?

Aggression in the workplace

The contribution the nurse makes to patient care is in collaboration with others, whether directly or indirectly. The effectiveness of this team is essential to patient care; however, the team's efficiency and morale can be undermined if there is little mutual level of respect and collegiality between team members. Sometimes, aggression and bullying are evident in these team endeavours. Bullying is, unfortunately, commonplace in many organisations and professions. Nursing is particularly susceptible to bullying because of the many stressors in the working environment. The impact can be significant, including depression and lower levels of job satisfaction. This could escalate into significant problems for both the individual and the organisation. Leaving the profession is a solution for some, but this has a cost – both personally and financially. Educating and training new nurses is time-consuming and expensive. Therefore, to lose nurses because of unnecessary behaviour by others exacts a high cost not only from the organisation but also from the individual nurse who has been the target of bullying behaviours.

Workplace bullying

workplace bullying: repeated aggressive behaviour against work colleagues

Workplace bullying is a common occurrence that appears to be worse than ever if media reports are any gauge. It could be that people are more aware of it, and some victims won't simply 'put up with it', so reporting of bullying is now more common. Lutgen-Sandvik and Tracy's (2012, p. 5) definition of workplace bullying reflects the dire situation for a person who is the target of bullying:

> Workplace bullying is a toxic combination of unrelenting emotional abuse, social ostracism, interactional terrorizing, and other destructive communication that erodes organizational health and damages employee well-being.

Bullying usually takes place over a long period of time, and its impacts can vary, depending on the emotional makeup of the victim. A power disparity is often an element of bullying in the workplace (Lutgen-Sandvik, Tracy & Alberts, 2007). This power disparity could be a result of the status differences in the organisation, or it could develop over time even if the perpetrator and the target are at the same level – that is, the perpetrator has gained psychological power over the target.

Chan-Mok, Caponecchia and Winder (2014) provide some examples of bullying behaviours in the workplace:

- undue public criticism
- name-calling, insults or intimidation
- social or physical isolation
- overwork (such as impossible deadlines, undue disruptions)
- destablilisation and undermining behaviour, such as not giving credit, assigning meaningless tasks, setting people up to fail, reminding people of their mistakes, removing responsibility without cause
- spreading malicious rumours and gossip
- assignment of duties that are obviously unfavourable to a particular individual
- withholding or denying access to necessary information, consultation or other resources.

A 'one off' incident may not be a problem, but when there is a sustained campaign of bullying, it can have serious psychological and physical health impacts.

Inventories applied specifically to the Australian hospital context have been developed by Hutchinson et al. (2008); these reflect some of the following elements:

- attacks on competence and reputation (for example, questioning competence and damaging reputation through false allegations)
- personal attacks (for example, belittling a person in front of others, threatening behaviour)
- attacks through work tasks (for example, excessive scrutinising and being assigned belittling work not reflecting skill level).

Workplace bullying is common in the nursing sector, and victims cope with it in various ways; this often means they do nothing. Cooper et al. (2009) found that 72 per cent of nursing students who experienced bullying did nothing to intervene to stop the behaviour. Instead, they put up barriers to distance themselves from the problem and pretended not to see what was happening. Cooper et al. (2009) suggest that nursing students have ineffective means of coping with bullying, and that this is a threat to their professional development. Therefore, it is useful for nursing students to educate themselves about the psychological and structural motivators that combine to create a climate of bullying. This knowledge will mentally prepare them to deal with situations more assertively and confidently.

Motivation for bullying

Like all human interaction, people who bully others have different motivations for their behaviour. To stereotype the bully in one particular way may be short-sighted, as there could be many factors in their lives that have led them to this point. One of the primary reasons a bully targets someone is to gain control. The bully tries to assert a level of power and authority over the target. It may be their need to manipulate others to get what they want or a fear of exposure or being vulnerable if they appear too easygoing. Personality flaws are another reason, and in extreme cases, psychopathic tendencies – including being 're-pulsively' charming (Murray, 2009) – are present. Reasons for bullying range from the benign, such as a lack of awareness, to the aggressive, such as seeking power, and pathological, as in personality disorders.

Impact of bullying on the individual

Bullying can sometimes be tolerated by nurse managers because the bully may be a reliable, efficient, competent clinician and is valued as a member of the team because of these characteristics. Tolerance of the dysfunctional bullying behaviours can become the norm, and be accepted, because the bully continues to contribute positively to the team. Ceravolo et al. (2012) advise that some nurses are unaware of the impact they have on others in the workplace. However, unless there is some kind of recognition or self-awareness, and ultimately a change in behaviour, the impact on the victim is not diminished by the intent of the perpetrator. The onus is on *all* nurses to challenge this ignorance if workplace bullying rates are to be reduced.

At best, the impact of bullying can be mild and transient, depending on the dynamics of the situation. At worst, the impact can be profound and ongoing. There is a range of symptoms and consequences of bullying. These include *psychological* consequences such as fear, vulnerability, loss of self-esteem, anxiety, sleeplessness, depression, demoralisation, panic attacks and even suicide (Hutchinson et al., 2008). The psychological pain can lead to *physical problems*, including psychosomatic illnesses such as dizziness, stomach aches, headaches, backaches, chronic fatigue and insomnia. High blood pressure and even cardiovascular problems have been identified as possible consequences (Moayed et al., 2006). The combination of psychological and physical manifestations can lead to adverse consequences, not just for the target and their family but also for the team, the patients and the organisation.

Impact of bullying on the organisation

Nurse managers sometimes dismiss bullying as an overreaction by the victim. Managers might explain the circumstances away as the bully is 'just having a bad day'. This lack of understanding can leave the target isolated and angry, and because what they report is disregarded, it may also have other consequences. Absenteeism can increase, as the target may need sick leave to recover from ill-health created by the situation or as respite from the abuse. The longer-term problem for the organisation is that the situation will become intolerable, and some nurses will leave their jobs as a result. This is a costly consequence for the employer. The aged care sector is particularly susceptible, as there is a shortage of nurses; therefore nurse managers need to address workplace bullying and implement zero-tolerance policies (Rodwell & Demir, 2012). (See discussion below on zero tolerance.)

There are also hidden costs to the organisation. With every bullying complaint or situation, there can be a great deal of time invested in exploring the problem, counselling and mediation, and dismissal processes. If the complaints develop into legal proceedings, this can further consume valuable financial and organisational resources along with the personal resources of the bully and their target.

Strategies to overcome bullying

Zero tolerance

There is a consistent theme in nursing literature of zero tolerance of bullying. Human resource departments in many organisations have created strong policies and procedures to counter bullying. In the healthcare context, policies and guidelines such as zero tolerance, prohibitive statements about violence and bullying and codes of practice have been put in place to make early identification, management and prevention possible (Hutchinson, 2009). There should be consequences for bullying, no matter what the circumstances. Enacting the zero-tolerance policies and procedures could solve an immediate problem, and could alert others to the consequences of bullying behaviour; however, whether the circumstances are revealed often depends on the skill of the investigators and strength of the victim. Hutchinson (2006, quoted in Hutchinson, 2009, pp. 149–50) confirms this, saying 'it appears in-house approaches to dealing with reports of bullying have little effect in reducing its occurrence with evidence reports are minimised, ignored, or denied'. Therefore, zero tolerance may not be an effective strategy when the facts are not acknowledged in the first place.

There are systemic problems within organisations that can actually reward bullying behaviour. Lutgen-Sandvik and Tracy (2012) argue that while bullying occurs between two people, the over-arching problem is that organisations perpetuate the problem by culturally accepting bullying. As noted above, the bully might be perceived as being very valuable to the workforce, and investigators could have loyalty to the bully. Human resource policies, with their structured lines of communication and delegation of authority, often identify the clinical unit manager as the person who reports bullying. However, the manager is also responsible for adequately staffing the unit to deliver the service safely. If the bully is essential to the unit workforce, then the manager can be conflicted, and might attempt other strategies before enacting policy. In this circumstance, they may take the opportunity to downplay the impact on the target. If the bully is successfully managing organisational goals, managers may be reluctant to implement a zero-tolerance penalty because they may be losing a 'star' employee. Employees are more likely to be rewarded when they obtain desired outcomes and performance outputs; that is, they make the right connection with their audience.

People in positions of power are likely to be more concerned with furthering their own interests by achieving their desired goals, rather than concentrating on addressing the welfare of their employees. Organisations that are rule- and outcomes-oriented are more likely to attribute blame for workplace problems to individuals, and treat bullying as a personality conflict rather than as a reflection of organisational practices – that is, acknowledging that there may be problems that are exacerbated by the structure of the workplace, or in its processes and procedures. In this context, bullying may be seen as a normal part of the way the workplace functions, and raising a grievance about bullying may result in further victimisation (Hutchinson & Hurley, 2013). Therefore, solutions like zero tolerance to bullying cannot always be entrusted to management.

Restorative justice

Hutchinson (2009, p. 149) argues that restorative approaches to bullying may be more effective than in-house approaches. The restorative justice approach involves the parties and representatives of the community (in this case, nursing) coming together to address the problem and rebuild social relationships. This approach removes the hierarchical power structure and gives the individuals involved a chance to rebuild relationships. This is achieved through cooperation to identify the causative factors. The impact of the bullying behaviour is openly discussed. In this way, the aim is that the target is less isolated and the bully is more sensitised to the impact on both the victim and the team. Clarifying the contributing factors encourages analysis of the problem and enables solutions to be considered.

The key elements of the restorative justice approach, adapted from Hutchinson (2009), include the following:

- The facilitator is the mediator of the discussion, who shares concern for the harmed individual/s. Participants are asked to reveal what they know about the situation and whether they have taken an active or passive role.
- The bullying behaviour is challenged, but in a respectful way.

- Members are responsible for curbing dominating or abusive language, and make sure individuals are not compromised by the words of others.
- Members take responsibility for ensuring that the perpetrator acknowledges and takes responsibility for their actions and the harmful impact on the victim.
- The perpetrator is asked what they can do to make up for the harm caused and to outline what steps they will take to make sure it does not happen again.
- Participants should *not* focus on blame, but rather on constructive strategies to change the situation.
- Members make the necessary commitment to help the perpetrator reach their goals to compensate for the behaviour.
- If members of the group have colluded in the bullying, they make a commitment to refrain from such behaviour in the future.

This is collegial and a less psychologically exacting process than other policy-driven organisational strategies or legal solutions. Supporting each member to be more self-aware and control their behaviour establishes more positive expectations for future interactions.

Cognitive reappraisal

The target could recover some psychological edge by observing the bully. Gaining knowledge of the personality and personal circumstances of the bully can help the target to distance themselves from the bully. An informed perspective of the bully helps to reframe the problem, and this *cognitive reappraisal* can change the dynamics, including the vulnerability of the target. According to Wilkins (2014), attribution theorists suggest it is the interpretation of bullying as stressful that causes stress, not the actual bullying behaviours. This is difficult to believe when experiencing the bullying 'storm'. However, the author states that because it is difficult to make sense of bullying when you view the world as a 'just world', cognitive reappraisal can help alter attributions about the bullying, and this can improve self-esteem and confidence in the target. Wilkins (2014) also argues that humour can be a powerful coping mechanism. By using humour, victims can distance themselves and reflect on the situation. Wilkins (2014, p. 293) maintains that, 'Laughter itself is incompatible with anger and negative affective states', and that humour will reduce the potential for aggression in the workplace. On a practical level, Murray (2009) offers some useful strategies to help protect against bullying (see Table 6.1).

TABLE 6.1 *A range of strategies to help minimise bullying of nurses*

HOW NURSES CAN PROTECT THEMSELVES	WHAT NURSING CO-WORKERS CAN DO
From the factors already presented, nurses can recognise when bullying exists. Individuals may be told repeatedly that they are not victims.	Colleagues should be prepared to acknowledge and challenge the bullying behaviour using unconditional positive regard as the foundation for professional communication. This technique can encourage the bully to retreat, or to recognise that the bullying behaviour has been exposed.
Nurses should seek support and counselling services to help deal with what can be an overwhelming experience. Once the crisis is over, practise reflexivity.	A fellow nurse should provide support for the target immediately following the episode.
Nurses must self-monitor their health to ascertain whether there are symptoms such as anxiety, loss of sleep and eating disorders as a result of bullying behaviour.	The incident should be brought immediately to the attention of the supervisor or management.
Nurses need to understand their rights by becoming familiar with organisations that can help.	Co-workers should not side with the bully. There may be some short-term gain, but the greater ethical cost is not worth it. The observer should not encourage bullying under any circumstances.
Nurses must be knowledgeable about workplace policies and procedures relating to bullying and procedures.	Staff should offer to attend meetings as witnesses when the bully meets with the target.
A bullying victim should document all incidents of bullying, including date, time, site of occurrence and witnesses.	Staff should support the target by providing written statements, documentation and/or sworn testimony at legal proceedings.
Nurses should be prepared for the fact that the organisation's management or senior leaders may not support them in favour of personal and professional interests.	
Legal assistance may be necessary if other avenues fail.	

Source: Adapted from Murray (2009)

Education

Preventative measures may be more effective than zero tolerance, and less complicated than managing bullying behaviour. In an extensive project by Ceravolo et al. (2012), it was found that having workshops on strengthening communication proved to be an effective strategy for addressing bullying and conflict issues. The workshops were based on making nurses aware of the problem and their role in it. Assertiveness, self-awareness and non-verbal communication were elements of the program. Nurse managers were educated to act as role models exhibiting behavioural expectations. Ceravolo et al. (2012) found that active participation in communication workshops helped to raise awareness of the problem, and led to a reduction in the turnover of staff. Some nurses unaware of their behaviour or its impact on their colleagues and communication education can increase awareness and result in significant improvements in attitudes and behaviour.

The last resort

In recent years, some promising research and projects have emerged to help arrest bullying in the nursing context; however, there may be some situations where strategies do not work because the bully may not be a willing participant for change or because the targets cannot make people believe them. This goes back to the power imbalance, and sometimes the options are limited. Like most things in life, there are model solutions; however, if the parties involved are unwilling to participate openly and fairly, the process will be stalled. Alberts, Martin and Nakayama (2007, p. 296) argue that in some circumstances the low-power person may not be able to be heard. They assert:

> Obliging, or accommodating to the bully's demands, may be the only strategy if one wishes to remain in the organization. Withdrawing may be an option if one is willing to leave, and targets report that leaving the organization was the most effective, and often only, solution to the problem. Competing typically is not a useful strategy; it only intensifies the bully's abusive behaviour.

This is a discouraging outcome, given the emerging research on the effectiveness of communication education. Relenting may soon be the extreme exception.

Summary

Nurses have special obligations to be professional communicators. As such, they need to analyse their communication styles and be self-aware. This can be achieved by adopting reflective practices that can enhance self-concept. They also need to understand the importance of assertion in protecting patients' rights and themselves in bringing about resolutions to problems without alienating others. Understanding the modes of communication and the issues related to misinterpreting non-verbal cues can help to promote more effective techniques and styles of interpersonal interaction. These skills also can be used to analyse and address situations that place nurses at risk, particularly in terms of bullying. Organisational responses to bullying can often be inadequate in diminishing the problem of workplace bullying. Individuals who develop the strategies suggested in the chapter have a better chance of effectively handling situations where communication is a significant aspect.

Discussion and critical thinking questions

6.1 Do you think you are a self-aware person? If so, is this linked to reflective practice and does it improve your self-esteem and thus your self-concept? If not, why not?

6.2 Why is non-verbal communication so difficult to interpret in some situations?

6.3 Do you think that you may have inadvertently displayed bullying behaviours in your life? If so, how would you change such behaviours now?

6.4 List the health service policies and processes that are available to assist in this situation.

Learning extension

Think about a situation in which you have been involved that left you feeling comfortable or happy with the outcome – for example, a group assignment or organising a study group. Recall the way you communicated. Using the list of non-verbal communication modes in this chapter, write your thoughts about what you did well during the encounter. Consider how you can apply these strengths in the clinical setting to improve your therapeutic communication.

Further reading

Glass, N. (2010). *Interpersonal relating: Health care perspectives in communication, stress and crisis*. Melbourne: Palgrave Macmillan.

References

Alberts, J.K., Martin, J.N. & Nakayama, T.K. (2007). *Human communication in society*. Upper Saddle River, NJ: Pearson Education.

Arnold, E.C. & Underman Boggs, K. (2011). *Interpersonal relationships: Professional communication skills for nurses*. St Louis, MS: Elsevier.

Ceravolo, D.J., Schwartz, D.G., Foltz-Ramos, K.M. & Castner, J. (2012). Strengthening communication to overcome lateral violence. *Journal of Nursing Management*, 20: 599–606.

Chan, E.A., Jones, A. & Wong, K. (2013). The relationships between communication, care and time are intertwined: A narrative enquiry exploring the impact of time on registered nurses' work. *Journal of Advanced Nursing*, 69(9): 2020–9.

Chan-Mok, J.O., Caponecchia, C. & Winder, C. (2014). The concept of workplace bullying: Implications from Australian workplace health and safety law. *Psychiatry, Psychology and Law*, 21(3): 442–6.

Cooper, J.R.M., Walker, J.T., Winters, K., Williams, R., Askew, R. & Robinson, J.C. (2009). *Journal in Educational Research*, 19(3): 212–26.

Dempsey, J., Hillege, S. & Hill, R. (2014). *Fundamentals of nursing and midwifery: A person-centred approach to care*. Sydney: Lippincott Williams & Wilkins.

Devenny, B. & Duffy, K. (2013). Person-centred reflective practice. *Art and Science*, 28: 37–43.

Geller, S.M. (2012). *Therapeutic presence: A mindful approach to effective therapy*. Washington, DC: American Psychological Association.

Glass, N. (2010), *Interpersonal relating. Health care perspectives in communication, stress and crisis*. Melbourne: Palgrave Macmillan.

Happ, M.B., Garrett, K., DiVirgilio Thomas, D., Tate, J., George, E., Houze, M., Radtke, J. & Sereika, S. (2011). Nurse–patient communication interactions in the intensive care unit. *American Journal of Critical Care Online Now*, 20(2): e28–e40.

Haskard, K.B., Williams, S.L., DiMatteo, M.R., Heritage, J. & Rosenthal, R. (2008). The provider's voice: Patient satisfaction and the content-filtered speech of nurses and physicians in primary medical care, *Journal of Nonverbal Behaviour*, 32: 1–20.

Hillege, S., Hardy, J. & Glew, P. (2014). Communication. In J. Dempsey, S. Hillege & R. Hill (eds), *Fundamentals of nursing and midwifery – a person-centred approach to care*. Philadelphia: Lippincott Williams & Wilkins, pp. 114–39.

Hodge, A.N. & Marshall, A.P. (2007). Violence and aggression in the emergency department: A critical care perspective. *Australian Critical Care*, 20(2): 61–7.

Hutchinson, M. (2009). Restorative approaches to workplace bullying: Educating nurses towards shared responsibility. *Contemporary Nurse*, 32(1–2): 147–55.

Hutchinson, M. & Hurley, J. (2013). Exploring leadership capability and emotional intelligence as moderators of workplace bullying. *Journal of Nursing Management*, 21: 553–62.

Hutchinson, M., Wilkes, L., Vickers, M. & Jackson, D. (2008). The development and validation of a bullying inventory for the nursing workplace. *Nurse Researcher*, 15(2): 19–29.

International Council of Nurses (ICN) (2013). *Scope of nursing practice*. Retrieved 20 November 2014 from <http://www.icn.ch/images/stories/documents/publications/position_statements/B07_Scope_Nsg_Practice.pdf>.

Luft, J. (1984). *Group processes: An introduction to group dynamics*, 3rd edn. Houston, TX: Mayfield.

Lutgen-Sandvik, P. & Tracy, S.J. (2012). Answering five key questions about workplace bullying: How communication scholarship provides thought leadership for transforming abuse at work. *Management Communication Quarterly*, 26(1): 3–47.

Lutgen-Sandvik, P., Tracy, S.J. & Alberts, J.K. (2007). Burned by bullying in the American workplace: Prevalence, perception, degree and impact. *Journal of Management Studies*, 44(6): 837–62.

Maier-Lorentz, M. (2008). Transcultural nursing: Its importance in nursing practice. *Journal of Cultural Diversity*, 15(1):37–43.

Mann, K., Gordon, J. & Macleod, A. (2009). Reflection and reflective practice in health professions education: A systematic review. *Advances in Health Sciences Education: Theory and Practice*, 14(4): 495–621.

Moayed, F.A., Daraishen, N., Shell, R. & Salem, S. (2006). Workplace: A systematic review of risk factors and outcomes. *Theoretical Issues in Ergonomics Science*, 7(3): 311–27.

Moyle, W., Parker, D. & Bramble, M. (2014). *Care of older adults: A strengths-based approach*. Melbourne: Cambridge University Press.

Murray, J.S. (2009). Workplace bullying in nursing: A problem that can't be ignored, *Medsurg, Nursing*, 19(5): 273–6.

Nursing and Midwifery Board of Australia (NMBA) (2006). *National competency standards for the registered nurse*. Sydney: NMBA.

——(2013). *Framework for assessing national competency standards*. Sydney: NMBA.

Nursing Council of New Zealand (2014). *Code of conduct*. Retrieved 20 November 2014 from <http://www.nursingcouncil.org.nz/Nurses/Code-of-Conduct>.

Rodwell, J. & Demir, D. (2012). Psychological consequences of bullying for hospital and aged care nurses. *International Nursing Review*, 59(4): 539–46.

Stein-Parbury, J. (2014). *Patient and person: Interpersonal skills in nursing*, 5th edn. Retrieved 20 November 2014 from <http://www.usq.eblib.com.au.ezproxy.usq.edu.au/patron/FullRecord.aspx?p=1723767>.

Wilkins, J. (2014). The use of cognitive reappraisal and humour as coping strategies for bullied nurses. *International Journal of Nursing Practice*, 20: 283–92.

Woloshynowych, L.J., Davis, R., Brown, R. & Vincent, C. (2007). Communication patterns in a UK emergency department. *Annals of Emergency Medicine*, 50(40): 407–13.

World Health Organization (2014). *Health workforce – nursing and midwifery*. Retrieved 20 November 2014 from <http://www.who.int/hrh/nursing_midwifery/en>.

7 Digital skills in healthcare practice

Clint Moloney and Helen Farley

Learning objectives

- Become familiar with developments in digital technologies in both education and healthcare settings.

- Become acquainted with some of the main debates around the introduction of emerging technologies into education and healthcare settings.

- Learn about some of the digital tools available for learning, research, collaboration and career development.

- Become aware of the risks and challenges associated with the use of online, digital technologies in education and healthcare settings.

- Understand some of the key terms associated with the discussion around digital technologies for study and use in the workplace.

Key terms

- Critical digital literacy
- Digital literacies
- Information literacy
- Intranet
- Media literacy
- Multiliteracies
- Social media

Introduction

The healthcare industry is rapidly evolving in tandem with a demand for increased flexibility in the delivery of education in our fast-paced society. As a result, the passive reception of content by students, delivered by an expert from the front of the class, is becoming an increasingly redundant method. Students now have always-on connectivity, facilitating widespread access to online materials (Collier, Gray & Ahn, 2011). Programs such as nursing are often offered in an external, online delivery mode (Wright, 2013). Due to an increasingly ageing population, healthcare is by far one of the fastest-growing industries, and graduate job seekers choosing to enter healthcare will need to ensure that they have developed sound **digital literacies**, particularly as they apply to professional communication. It is imperative that students develop and leverage emerging communication technologies as part of their portfolio prior to seeking employment (Clark, 2009; Hargittai & Litt, 2013).

> **digital literacies:** the skill set needed to effectively use digital technologies in order to access, understand and participate in the digital world

Context of digital skills in healthcare practice

Research reveals that the more a hospital embraces digital technologies the better off its patients will be (Govindan et al., 2010). The evidence indicates there are likely to be fewer cases of patient harm and fewer complications associated with document management. Unfortunately, only a small percentage of hospitals and doctors' offices are currently embracing digital technologies, and the majority of healthcare providers lag far behind other more developed healthcare settings in implementing these innovations (Govindan et al., 2010; Wetterneck et al., 2006). However, researchers, legislators and digital technology experts hope this change will come about over the next decade, with some strong investment in infrastructure. Such investments should enable the adoption of healthcare education technologies such as remote access systems, telehealth, electronic health records and patient tracking systems and, most importantly, staff and patient education in these areas (Gill, Gill & Young, 2013; Gyurko & Ullmann, 2012). Due to the rapid advancement of technologies that have enabled the gathering and sharing of information, and real-time communications in healthcare, the healthcare professionals of tomorrow (who are learning today) essentially need to become experts in the use of these technologies. For example, nursing students studying today need to familiarise themselves with digital technologies to ensure their application in the clinical context is safe, effective and user-friendly. The digital skills learnt today will save time in the workplace, streamlining processes and expediting communication (Dudding, 2009). By way of example, though telehealth is more common than it once was, certain technical, social and infrastructural barriers prevent its more common use in nursing. As restrictions around nursing licensure change to accommodate changing practices and technologies, telehealth use by nurse practitioners will only increase. In order to move forward, nursing students need to embrace these communication technologies as part of their professional development.

Telehealth can also play a key role in the ongoing training of nursing students engaging in clinical placement. The technology allows training and technical support for the use of distance learning while nursing students are on clinical placement. Greater support at the bedside for students has never been more possible than now. Mobile applications such as FaceTime or Facebook, and free communication tools like Skype, can now provide students with remote support for their learning needs (Gassert, 2000; Nguyen, Zierler & Nguyen, 2011).

Mobile and online communications: Distance learning strategies

Online learning facilitates students' abilities to learn at their own convenience and at their own pace (Hamilton & Friesen, 2013; Sawyer & Howard, 2007). Some would argue that the physical separation from fellow learners and teachers may result in a reduction in communication and important social interactions, and the development of an uncertain sense of attachment to a community of learners. Researchers argue that these feelings of detachment may affect a student's motivation, and could lead to reduced performance, more dissatisfaction and increased attrition (Horn, 2013; Kelland, 2011). Hence those opposed to online learning would suggest that face-to-face interaction can positively influence learners' motivation, active participation and interest in learning (Thompson & Lynch, 2003). However, these theories fail because they do not consider the options for flexibility that online technologies afford. Online technologies do offer a sound platform for personal interaction, with the capacity to facilitate effective communication (Gyurko & Ullmann, 2012). In addition, face-to-face learning is not an option for many rural and remote learners. For some learners, there is no alternative but to participate online and at a distance (McLeod & Barbara, 2005).

Research that has focused on online communication in education has generally centred around the generation of personal interactions, reading and writing capabilities, or the effects of online learning on communication (Wright, 2013). This research has demonstrated that online communication tends to lead to more balanced contributions than face-to-face engagement, with less dominance by highly opinionated personalities (Gill, Gill & Young, 2013; Hamilton & Friesen, 2013; Warschauer, 2001). Participation in communication is an essential ingredient of learning, and introverted personalities who are less likely to contribute in face-to-face discussions are more likely to participate in, and make valuable contributions to, discussion in an online environment (Yan, 2013). This gives digital communication platforms a distinct advantage when compared with traditional, didactic systems of learning. There is clear evidence that reading and writing skills can improve when students are also asked to engage with online learning materials. Well-validated research indicates that this arises because students take more pride in their work when posting something on an online platform (McAllister & Watkins, 2012; Roper, 2007). The impact of online learning can be measured by the extent to which it improves access to information, and therefore the generation of knowledge. The online delivery of programs and courses allows students to participate, irrespective of their geographical location. A message, activity or piece of content can reach a wide audience in a matter of seconds (Gill, Gill & Young, 2013; McLeod & Barbara, 2005). Often people seek expert opinions, viewpoints and points of clarity on given topics or best practices. Ready access is the key to keeping people engaged, and mobile communication via online media allows this (Collier, Gray & Ahn, 2011).

It can be difficult to stay up to date with the latest information. Even the best-intentioned student can forget how to complete every procedure, or remember all the processes and policies needed to work in a hospital or other healthcare setting. Mobile devices have the potential to revolutionise the way nurses learn and to enable them to remain up to date with the latest information. In 2014, some 70 per cent of Australians owned a smartphone or a tablet device, with nearly one-third of people owning both. The average Australian adult owned four mobile devices (Deepend, 2014). Ownership rates in New Zealand are comparably high: in 2012, 60 per cent of New Zealand adults owned smartphones and 19 per cent owned tablets (News, 2013).

Because mobile devices are easily carried on the person, they serve as portals to online information. Textbooks and articles can readily be accessed, searched and read using mobile devices – particularly tablets (Duffy, 2012). YouTube or Vimeo videos can be viewed showing examples of processes and procedures (Clifton & Mann, 2011). By using mobile devices for learning, educators are leveraging the skills and technologies students already have, making them more likely to be adopted for study and in the workplace.

Emerging learning technologies

Those in favour of mobile and online learning technologies tend to believe that they offer a learner the ability to interact synchronously or asynchronously with their teachers and peers, in real time at any hour of the day, regardless of time zones. This can also mean that the teacher does not always need to be present for learning to occur; rather, students can engage with each other at their own convenience. Although communication with a teacher may be delayed, it can still occur, and an individual's learning needs can be met (Bozalek et al., 2013; Herrington & Parker, 2013). University academics often make use of online communication and learning strategies, inclusive of discussion forums or real-time virtual classrooms. The virtual classroom can enable group communication and facilitate effective discussion, even allowing for group work in rooms within the virtual classroom before reconvening class discussions (Martin, Parker & Allred Oyarzun, 2013; Taras et al., 2013). Researchers are also working on remote-access systems that enable a high fidelity of learning, such as emulated intravenous pumps. These offer learners basic through to complex learning scenarios that have been shown to be as effective as face-to-face training (Bowtell et al., 2012). In this way, face-to-face practical or clinical sessions can be emulated online.

YouTube, multimedia and open learning resources in the form of short snippets or lectures, simulations, animations and virtual world scenarios provide academics and students with a variety of teaching and learning tools (Gill, Gill & Young, 2013). These can be applied and adapted to learning needs in various ways, ensuring personal learning styles are not neglected. Many of these platforms offer the learner a chance to effectively practise the art of communication prior to engaging in real-world scenarios (Bowtell et al., 2012).

Open online learning resources can help students who have never fully mastered key concepts, or who have perhaps forgotten them (Bowtell et al., 2012), to learn. They provide options for students who have struggled to follow or engage in classroom tutorials (Gill, Gill & Young, 2013). Even textbooks are changing to incorporate video and audio clips, animations and rich graphics. These textbooks are becoming more interactive, allowing both instructors and students to annotate, add or change material – including interactive assessment questions and feedback. These electronic texts are, of course, accessible via smartphones, tablets, e-readers and other mobile devices (Brown, 2012; Rockinson-Szapkiw et al., 2013).

Case study

A university's nursing course has taken its entire program to an external online student cohort to help capture a wider population of students into the program and to ensure strong, sustainable enrolment numbers.

Critical reflection

》 How will students ensure equitable and comparable access to effective communication in the online system, compared with communicating with their lecturer face to face?

》 How will students seek clarity on content?

》 If a student is struggling with content, how will they be able to ensure they receive support from the teaching team or other students?

Digital learning as a substitution process

Time is always a limiting factor when it comes to learning opportunities – or, more importantly, *exposure* to the best learning opportunities. This particularly occurs when students need to acquire certain competencies in a given timeframe (Bowtell et al., 2012; Miranda & Lima, 2013). In a typical nursing program, most students have limited exposure to simulated patient scenarios or real clinical experience. The capacity to learn and test effective communication skills is therefore somewhat limited. It is imperative that trainee health professionals get adequate exposure to high-fidelity communication scenarios involving patient interaction, as well as interaction with other healthcare professionals. This can occur using several frameworks (Peters, 2004) – for example, ISBAR (Introduction, Situation, Background, Assessment and Recommendation) is a well-known tool used to communicate patient issues with colleagues (see Chapter 2 and Chapter 4). It was originally developed in the military to ensure effective communication of key issues from one person to another. By using the tool, a person can better plan their communication, making it clear and precise for the end receiver and thereby reducing the likelihood of misunderstanding (Brindley & Reynolds, 2011). It is particularly effective for ensuring that all key messages are summarised, particularly if a health professional requires some urgent action regarding a patient. Another valuable tool is PACE (Probe, Alert, Challenge and Emergency). This is valuable when a healthcare professional believes a patient may be at a significant risk due to the actions of another healthcare professional. Using graded assertiveness, a healthcare professional can learn to PACE their way through some effective communication in order to prevent patient harm (Brindley & Reynolds, 2011).

In real-world training environments, there is often minimal exposure to the types of situations in which nurse or other health professional students can develop and make use of such communication tools. However, digital learning environments such as virtual clinical settings can provide a platform for repetitive exposure to conflict scenarios or challenging situations that require effective communication. This enables a student to better develop communication competence and confidence. As another example, simulated nursing labs offer an effective means for students to practise communication with patients regarding everyday procedures such as wound management and medication administration (Bowtell et al., 2012).

The driving societal forces for online learning

Online teaching platforms are fast becoming more popular, with their use expanding well beyond the university sector and into the business and healthcare domains. Study within university climates that include remote training and instruction, and video web conferencing (Peters, 2004), can only become more popular. Together with the popularity of online learning, websites and innovative learning technologies are also being developed by academics to cater for the conversion to learning via distance modes. One of the major driving forces has been the changing expectations for academic learning in online learning environments. Applications with specific operations and purposes are also being created to cater for the increasing online demand and presence of students (Shen et al., 2013). These are being designed to aid learning, ensuring there is equivalence with traditional face-to-face models, while also matching the everyday social expectations of online **social media** (Macdonald, 2004).

social media: websites and applications that enable users to share content and participate in social networking

The sudden escalation in and popularity of social media applications have made it possible to create an environment that offers variety and flexibility. This means that modern students need to remain current and open to rapid change in learning systems. A variety of communication applications, such as practice labs, student self-checks, teacher lesson plans, social forums, virtual classrooms such as Blackboard Collaborate, chat and other forums enable effective communication with teaching staff. The modern student wants to balance family, work and study; the development and further refinement of innovative online systems and supporting applications is now making this desire a reality (Cui, Lockee & Meng, 2013).

Without the rapid evolution of these applications, online delivery might not have received the widespread endorsement it currently enjoys. Online applications offer a conducive environment for students and their teachers, as well as trainees and instructors. Such applications help with the creation and management of flexible lesson planning, access to and management of digital library resources, readily available and cyclical student feedback with online surveys, electronic assignment submission and online examination (Cui, Lockee & Meng, 2013). Access to internationally relevant content is now both a key feature and a driving demand from students. The internet has opened up the ability to rapidly acquire information and synthesise it into something meaningful (Keengwe, Adjei-Boateng & Diteeyont, 2013; Shen et al., 2013).

Digital literacies and learning inequalities

In online learning environments, students need to be able to identify, locate, evaluate and effectively use information for their own professional learning and personal improvement. This means they must be able to navigate a plethora of new and rapidly evolving technologies. We tend to think younger generations are like sponges, and generally adapt very quickly to new systems and applications. However, it is wrong to assume that every individual has the competency and capacity for such an adaptation. High school curricula still invest little energy into this new way of learning, and many school leavers are still not digitally literate (Beach et al., 2009; Cui, Lockee & Meng, 2013). Therefore, the university sector must formulate orientations that familiarise new students with the online environment (Roper, 2007).

The internet provides access to a staggering variety of information from online academic journals to practitioner blogs, YouTube videos, Facebook groups and websites of all descriptions. The problem is not a lack of information but rather determining which of these sources are reliable and credible. In the healthcare setting, using incorrect or out-of-date information can have significant consequences. The ability to search for, locate, evaluate and use the information needed is known as **information literacy** (Eisenberg, 2008). It is not enough to be able to use a

information literacy: a set of skills for searching for, locating, evaluating and using information

computer or mobile device. The modern practitioner needs to be able to apply those computing skills to address real-world situations and challenges, and to be able to locate the information that will help to solve those problems.

A number of attempts have been made to better define 'digital literacies' and their relationship to acquiring knowledge and skills. Other educational goals inclusive of traditional learning modes, such as computer training, library access and use, and clinical reasoning skills, relate to information literacy. The necessary digital literacies are evolving over time, and are essential tools to ensure social and academic well-being in a complex and rapidly evolving society (Macdonald, 2004).

Governments and educational institutions around the world need to challenge traditional methods of learning and embrace the flexibility and diversity that online systems and applications offer. In modern-day learning, there is a need to move away from the traditional learning of effective communication. Communicating online requires the development of quite specific skills, which might include knowing how to use videoconferencing, teleconferencing, opening and listening to Mp3 and Mp4 files, or something as simple as sending an email. It is imperative that a student entering the academic world learns and understands the etiquette of communicating via these tools (Duffy, 2012; Macdonald, 2004).

Media literacy

Very few healthcare students are exposed to online media as a tool for learning. This is surprising, given the potential to assist in the development of learners' critical thinking and creative abilities. The benefits of using online media in learning are that the information has no fixed location, no clear philosophy and no conclusive receivers. Online media are dependent on the erratic nature of news broadcasters and enable communication about what is currently topical and important to the learner. Often, very good case studies can come at timely points in the learning cycle to reinforce key messages. By using and interpreting the media, students are able to analyse, evaluate and generate messages in a vast array of media, genres and configurations. Students who are media literate stay informed about current and relevant events that affect their profession. This reveals current trends and issues within the healthcare sector, and can help generate timely reactions and solutions to minimise public outrage (Lukinbeal, 2014; Sur, Ünal & İşeri, 2014).

media literacy: the ability to decode, evaluate, analyse and produce messages in a wide variety of media formats

Media literacy is the ability to decode, evaluate, analyse and produce both print and electronic media (Aufderheide, 1992). Someone who is media literate should feel comfortable with all forms of media, from newspapers to social media, television and even internet search engines. Media can be a form of entertainment and a way of accessing culture – either our own or that of others. Media literacy is also critically important for learning. With so much media available in our society, the student needs to be able to critically analyse that form of media, gauging its quality and accuracy. This becomes very important when assessing the value of a medical aid or treatment that is being advertised (Koltay, 2011). Media literacy includes knowledge of when discretion with media is required – for example, to maintain patient privacy.

> Look at your current social media profile. How can it be leveraged to increase your professional profile?

> If you don't engage with social media, choose an appropriate platform to write about. Note down the elements you think would contribute towards a professional social media profile.

> If you have an account, you may want to implement these strategies.

Multiliteracies

Multiliteracies is a recent label that is used to reflect the ways in which people communicate with new technologies. Mobile phones and social media have created a shift in the way the English language is used, meaning a new 'literacy' must now be embraced. As an example, people now use emoticons to describe how they are feeling or use abbreviated terms that enable timely replies. In healthcare, these new forms of communication need to be incorporated into learning. Ubiquitous connectivity makes the world seem smaller, cultures have become intertwined and a mix of languages is giving rise to variations in the English language (Rowland et al., 2014; Tan & Guo, 2014).

multiliteracies: the skill set needed to create meaning in ways that are increasingly multimodal, and in which text interfaces with oral, visual, audio, gestural, tactile and spatial patterns of meaning

These variations, combined with the rapid evolution in technology and multimedia, have caused a sudden shift in communication. Today, text messaging via phones is not the only way to communicate. Text messages provide a way to interact with sounds and images, movies, posters, different websites and television programs. To survive and thrive, an individual needs to be familiar with these differing modes of communication, and know what it means to live in a multimedia world (Aufderheide, 1992; Sur, Ünal & İşeri, 2014).

Critical digital literacy

Critical digital literacy is necessary in order for all students to learn effectively in online environments. Students require the technological skills and confidence that enable effective access to, and navigation and use of, online information. With the evolution of digital learning platforms, curriculum design has now

critical digital literacy: digital literacies with a focus on critical thinking skills

become more complex, meaning multiple tools can be used to engage students in their own learning (Avila & Pandya, 2013). In nursing, teachers like to communicate with storytelling or situated practice. The benefit to the nursing student is that they can learn from realistic case studies, receiving high-fidelity learning experiences prior to engaging in the real world. This communicates the realities of healthcare, and enables the development of required clinical reasoning skills prior to students taking on real-life problems. Online engagement allows a student to repeatedly receive instruction, and this can build confidence in handling difficult or complex scenarios or tasks. Healthcare students need to build their perception skills – their ability to recognise non-verbal cues or hidden elements in the communication process. The concept of emotional intelligence is paramount, and online case studies or even patient communities can enable the development of better critical thinking processes, enhance perceptual skills and help students to discover their own emotional intelligence in perceiving when colleagues or patients need assistance. The development of critical digital literacies has the capacity to help transform practice. It can enable students to make connections with key concepts before entering the real world – something that can offer students safer and more confident practice (Avila & Pandya, 2013; Greene, Yu & Copeland, 2014).

Digital exclusion

Being digitally literate can create job opportunities through allowing flexibility when working remotely. Students with the right skill sets can receive a live lecture from the other side of the globe. With the emergence of cheaper forms of communication and increasing numbers of social network interactions, the development of online skills and knowledge has become paramount. If they fail to pay attention, students and their teachers can easily be left behind in the light of these rapidly changing innovations that make extensive use of the internet (Aleixo, Nunes & Isaias, 2012).

Digital inequality is a significant issue that, if left unrecognised, can mean diminished communication with a student or a patient in a healthcare setting. Individuals without access, appropriate skills or the right motivation and knowledge will miss out on the digital revolution. Access to information in order to learn, improve and remain engaged with the world is considered by many to be a human right. In this digital world, it is questionable whether printed newspapers will continue to exist; many believe it is almost inevitable that news will soon be accessed exclusively online or via broadcast media. This could potentially lead to further social isolation for particular individuals or communities. Research now shows a clear correlation between digital resource development and social exclusion. The reality is that individuals who are already disadvantaged and who possibly have the most to gain from digital communications are the least likely to know how to use it (Aleixo, Nunes & Asais, 2012; Wong et al., 2009).

For those studying to be part of the healthcare system, it is imperative to keep up with advances in digital technologies, as the future is likely to be increasingly digital. Electronic health records are more prevalent, radiology is now digitalised and medication charts will soon be in a digital format. Nurses and other health professionals need to be digitally literate, ready with the required skills and knowledge (McIntyre, McDonald & Racine, 2013; Wong et al., 2009).

Digital technology and learning outcomes

Evidence suggests that behaviours change when people interact with online technologies (Bowtell et al., 2012; McIntyre, McDonald & Racine, 2013). Much of the literature refers to readiness for learning. In nursing, this means that the right online preparation has occurred, enabling an individual to explore their own and others' lifelong learning requirements. Digital technologies have been shown to provide rich cognitive resources, which can have a profound effect on an individual's learning experience. As an example, research has shown that three-dimensional objects better stimulate the human visual system, and lead to high-recognition processes – particularly with clinical reasoning. Examples online include three-dimensional exploration of the human body or specific parts of the anatomy in a simulated environment (Sinha & Poggio, 1996).

Learning technologies have never been more affordable, and laptops, voice-recognition software or text-to-speech software can greatly assist students with learning deficits. Online gaming is making learning more engaging (and fun) for the participant, and evidence suggests that this type of learning engenders greater memory recall (Collier, Gray & Ahn, 2011). Technologies are enabling learners to fully benefit from flexible and optional learning platforms, meaning it is easier to cater to a person's individual learning style. In academia, online learning strategies may include the provision of written materials supported with audio-visual delivery and remote access to devices with which students can practise and apply learned materials; the previously mentioned remote access intravenous pump emulation is a good example (Sawyer & Howard, 2007).

Online safety

Many people have an online presence and enjoy using social media sites such as Facebook, Instagram or Twitter. They comment on blogs and news stories, share photos and music with friends, and even sign up for online dating. This kind of sharing is now commonplace, and can be a positive and enriching aspect of our lives. Even so, sometimes this sharing can go very wrong. The media are littered with reports of online scams, cyberbullying and identity theft. This danger generally comes from oversharing personal information over the internet with people whose identity can't be verified.

There are a number of ways in which these risks can be minimised. The most obvious is to use only a screen name or nickname online. Users of social media sites are often encouraged to share a picture of themselves, but a safer option would be to use a cartoon avatar or a picture of a favourite band. Users should not share too much private information via social media: they should never supply an email address, surname, phone number or home address. Where possible, profiles should be kept private and only shared with friends or family members.

It is important to remember that anything posted can be disseminated more widely than the user is aware. For that reason, students must be cautious about uploading images or creating posts that can portray them in an unprofessional or unflattering light. A digital footprint can surface many years after the original posts were made, and many employers now conduct social media searches of those they are interviewing or recruiting. A few indiscreet pictures from a party can potentially impact on a person's chance of securing a job. Users need to think twice before they post.

Privacy is becoming increasingly important as nurses and other health professionals take their mobile devices into the workplace. Mobile devices can be used to take photographs or videos, or to look up information. The diversity of apps enables users to do a wide variety of activities, with users able to post 'selfies' or pictures of co-workers direct to their Facebook page, for example. Care must be taken to respect the privacy of patients when using mobile devices. In April 2014, a picture-sharing app for doctors and nurses made the news for all the wrong reasons – the app allowed practitioners to share photos of lesions with other practitioners and enable discussion to aid diagnosis. The app did contain some tools to help conceal the identity of the patient; however, there was no compulsion to use them (Smith, 2014). With a little additional information, the patient could be identified from the pictures, and many doctors and academics expressed dismay at the lack of guidelines to ensure patient privacy and confidentiality.

Making digital technologies work for you

Old models of scholarship were based around solid artefacts. Journals were all paper based and university libraries were populated with hard copies of books. Students studying at a distance would have to submit requests for reference materials in a letter and those materials would be posted or copied, and sent to the student. The delivery system relied on an efficient postal system so students in regional, rural and remote areas were often at a significant disadvantage, as materials could take weeks to arrive.

With the arrival of the internet, the delivery models for these resources have changed. Though hard copies of journals and books still exist, university libraries are increasingly buying subscriptions to online journals, book series and databases so that any student with an internet connection can access a particular article or resource at a time convenient to them (Pearce et al., 2010). This is perhaps expressed best by Christine Borgman (2007, p. xix), who states, 'The internet lies at the core of an advanced scholarly information infrastructure to facilitate distributed, data and information-intensive collaborative research.' This may be in the form of data sets that are assembled by one research team then made available for others to use in new ways (Borgman, 2007).

Another way the internet is opening up scholarship is through Web 2.0 technologies such as blogs, and social media tools such as Twitter and SlideShare

(Dabbagh & Reo, 2011). These technologies allow discoveries and experimental results to be disseminated widely and quickly to both scholars and the general public (Pearce et al., 2010). These sources become important in rapidly changing fields in which the length of time between submission and publication of journal articles can sometimes be counted in years. Dissemination through social media substantially shortens those timeframes, but on the downside this material can lack the rigorous process of peer review. This is where media and information literacy become very important. Consumers of these sources must be able to weigh up the credibility and validity of the data, its methods of collection, its analysis and the conclusions drawn from it. There is no gatekeeper to ensure the quality of these sources, so great caution and discrimination must be exercised when choosing whether or not to accept the conclusions.

There are many ways to search the internet for information, yet the one most people use is the Google search engine. For academic writing, many people use Google Scholar to find articles. Google and Google Scholar can help unearth all sorts of information from a variety of places. They can help find websites, images, videos and news items. What is often forgotten is that Google is a multinational corporation that makes substantial profits from advertising and partnership deals. For that reason, Google has attracted considerable criticism for directing searches towards its own products and those of its partners (Hazan, 2013). A Google search will undoubtedly reveal much information; however, it may not be the best information for a particular need. It is always worth trying one or two other sources and comparing the results. Other popular search engines include Bing and Ixquick.

For reliable academic information, many university libraries have their own customised search engines, which will search the databases and journals to which they subscribe. Using this method has the added bonus that a student will be able to directly access the resources they find. If a student does not have access to this customised service, the next best thing to do is to search the general databases to which the university subscribes. Certain databases tend to focus on particular topics or disciplines, and most libraries will recommend databases for particular disciplinary areas.

No matter where a student searches for information, there are a few strategies to maximise the value of the search. To make searching more effective, it is best to use Boolean searches using the terms 'and', 'or' and 'not'. If 'and' is used, the search will reveal those sources that contain whatever term is linked by the 'and', which is useful because it helps to narrow the search. For example, a search for 'AIDS' may reveal many thousands of results, but the search

'AIDS and Africa' will reveal far fewer results. The term 'or' finds those sources that have either or both of the search terms. This is helpful when more results are needed or when something is known by more than one name. An example would be the search for 'croup or laryngotracheobronchitis'. The Boolean search term 'not' can help exclude results; it is used when a search turns up many results that aren't relevant. An example of this kind of search would be 'arthritis NOT rheumatoid'. By using just these three Boolean search terms, a search can be refined so only relevant results are returned.

Case study

A new graduate of the university's nursing program wants to create an online professional presence for himself in order to find work.

Critical reflection

›› Which tools will he use and why?

›› How will he ensure his profile remains safe, and how will he protect himself from identity theft?

›› What will he do about some unflattering photos of himself at a party that were posted to Facebook two years earlier? Are they likely to impact on his career?

Using digital literacy to improve the quality of your assessment pieces

Think about the latest piece of written assessment you submitted. Now you have learnt about digital technologies for study and in the workplace, how would you do this assessment differently, using the tools and techniques you've just learnt about?

Communication and collaboration

Digital technologies are providing many opportunities for communication and collaboration (Dabbagh & Kitsantas, 2011). This potential is being realised in someone's personal time. Phone calls are increasingly giving way to text messaging and instant messaging through social media apps (mobile applications), such as Facebook, Skype, WhatsApp and a range of others. Pictures are shared across devices and applications, and ubiquitous connectivity means that a friend or colleague is never far away, no matter what time of the day or night it is. These technologies can be harnessed for use in professional life, and have several advantages over more traditional forms of communication: they are instantaneous; they can remove the need for travel; a digital record can be made of the interaction; and it is generally very low in cost.

Teleconferencing once required the use of high-end technical equipment that was generally only found in business or on a university campus. Now teleconferencing can be accessed for free via a variety of social media platforms. Skype, Facebook, Google Hangouts and FaceTime all offer free teleconferencing, usually with other features such as screen sharing, text messaging and recording. These applications will work as long as each user has an account, access to a mobile device or computer, and reasonable internet access. Some applications, such as Skype, will allow others to join the conversation via a phone number.

Document-sharing applications such as Google Docs, Wikispaces or Office 360 allow multiple users to edit the same document at the same time. This is a boon for collaborative writing, even when writers are in different time zones or countries. These applications allow users to annotate their changes, or leave explanations or descriptions of changes for other users to see. Storage applications such as Google Drive or Dropbox can be used for sharing large files between collaborators (Lasater et al., 2012). This is another way to facilitate collaborative writing, with individual collaborators working asynchronously on a document, which is then synced to the version held in the storage app. All these applications can be accessed either via personal computers or via a range of mobile devices, including smartphones or tablets.

Learning through simulations

It is often not possible to see every possible medical emergency when doing a clinical placement. Some clinical emergencies remain relatively uncommon. To make sure a nursing student can experience a wide range of emergencies, virtual world simulations may be used. A virtual world is an internet-based social environment that persists even when the user is logged out. The user interacts with the environment via a motional 'avatar', a representation of the user. This avatar can communicate with others via voice chat or text chat. *Second Life* is the most popular virtual world, and many universities use this environment for learning and teaching (Farley, 2011). Simulations may supplement clinical placements and reduce the load on real clinicians supervising clinical placements (Chodos et al., 2010).

Virtual world simulations provide immediate feedback on the consequences of clinical reasoning decisions, and therefore reinforce appropriate decision-making processes. Simulations may feature automated virtual patients who are really artificial intelligence 'bots' (robots), which have the capacity to respond immediately and realistically to the variety of treatment options that might be administered by nursing students. Students can use simulations both synchronously and asynchronously, by themselves or collaboratively with other students and/or academics (McCallum, Ness & Price, 2011).

Career and identity management

Though students should be cautious when using social media, in order to ensure their identities are safe, the ability to disseminate information about themselves can help to promote their careers. For the scholar, there are social media sites that are designed specifically to help disseminate research (Giglia, 2011). There are three commonly used sites: academia.edu, ResearchGate and Mendeley. There is no cost associated with joining any of them. Scholars have the opportunity to upload papers, ask questions of colleagues and find collaborators, both within and outside their own institutions. If a student doesn't have access to a university library, these sites act as useful places to find full-text articles supplied by the people who wrote them.

Another useful site to help build a career profile is LinkedIn. LinkedIn allows a user to create a profile, describe their work and list their study history. It is also helpful when looking for a job. A user can indicate their availability and allow potential employers to connect with them. As with all social media, the user must be careful to protect their identity and not reveal too much personal information. They must also critically assess the contacts made through this medium. As with all social media, not everyone is who they appear to be. A user should always try to verify the identity of the person with whom they are communicating by other means.

Communication technologies for study and in the workplace

Nearly every university hosts a learning management system (LMS) that supports the student through a course or program (Dabbagh & Kitsantas, 2011). Even if a course is taught face to face, there is still usually a component that is available online through the LMS. There are several different kinds of LMSs: Moodle and Blackboard are the most common, but others include Sakai and Desire2Learn. All operate in a similar way: there is usually a virtual space or series of spaces where course materials are held, including lecture recordings, multimedia and readings. Discussion boards facilitate communication and collaboration between students and instructors. There is often a capacity for self-marking online quizzes or the ability to submit more substantial assessments such as assignments and essays. The LMS usually makes use of a range of Web 2.0-like tools such as wikis or blogs. The student who is familiar with using Web 2.0 tools and social media is unlikely to have much difficulty navigating the institutional LMS.

In the workplace, the LMS is sometimes used to deliver specific training to employees (Pandey & Pathak, 2014). If it is a large organisation, there is usually an **intranet**, a private computer network that uses protocols and software usually developed for the internet. Access to the intranet is usually restricted to employees of a company or government department. The intranet allows access to a range of documentation necessary for the consistent functioning of the company, so there may be access to policies and procedures, report and presentation templates, training modules and so on. Within this secure environment, patient logs, systems for incident reports and ongoing alerts can also be housed, allowing ready access for employees while keeping the information secure from those outside of the organisation (Welsh, 2012).

intranet: an organisation's private network, based on internet technology and accessed via the internet; usually protected from unauthorised access by firewalls

There may be discussion boards or instant messaging enabled within the intranet to allow easy communication between employees and to provide an alternative to email communication. In other cases, proprietary social media channels could be used. A common social media, instant messaging tool used within organisations is Yammer, which allows the formation of special-interest groups, or more general dissemination of short messages and information sharing within a company or department. BuddyPress is a similar tool that allows instant communication and the sharing of resources and links (Santos, Brogueira & Bernardino, 2014).

Electronic records and clinical documentation

The concept of computer-based patient records or continuity of care records (CCR) has been around since the 1990s. These terms gave way to Electronic Health Records (EHR), which describes the idea of a cross-institutional collection of information pertaining to an individual's medical treatment and overall health (Hoerbst & Ammenwerth, 2010). The individual acts as a partner in the process by accessing and adding to the record, in that way supporting their own care (Ball, Smith & Bakalar, 2006). EHRs are designed to bring information together and facilitate communication between clinicians in order to improve patient care (Lehnbom, Brien & McLachlan, 2014).

The Australian government rolled out eHealth records in July 2012, though the awareness and uptake remain relatively low (Lehnbom, Brien & McLachlan, 2014). The situation is more complicated in New Zealand, where there is not yet a common system and a number of health organisations have their own systems in place (Stiftung, 2009).

Though EHRs have the potential to save considerable time and money through an efficient sharing of patient data between clinicians, there remain significant potential pitfalls that must be considered. There is always the potential of inappropriate sharing and dissemination of patient data, and other breaches of confidentiality and privacy. Other issues identified include authorship ambiguities (particularly where patients are able to directly amend the documents), misleading histories, inadequate discharge summaries and miscommunications between clinicians and patients (Bernat, 2013). For the most part, these risks can be mitigated if appropriate measures are put in place, but this risk mitigation requires the providers of electronic health records systems to work closely with clinicians and other stakeholders to ensure an effective and secure system.

Remote patient management

One of the developments opened up by the rapid evolution of technologies and devices is the possibility of remote monitoring of patient health. This usually requires implanting devices into appropriate places under the skin of the patient. The advantages are numerous: it can remove the need for patients to travel to their clinician or hospital for monitoring, thereby saving time and travel costs, and decreasing the strain on hospital resources. Remote management of patients with cardiac diseases is becoming increasingly common, even for people fitted with devices such as pacemakers and implanted cardiac defibrillators. Through a simple computer hook-up, clinicians are able to download data including electrograms, and access information about remote and recent cardio arrhythmic and haemodynamic events (Reynolds, Murray & Germany, 2008). As technology becomes increasingly sophisticated, the potential for programming and adjusting these devices at a distance becomes more feasible. Much research is being directed towards the use of chemical and physiological sensors that will allow the monitoring of chronic and acute illnesses (Reynolds, Murray & Germany, 2008).

Summary

The past decades have brought exciting advancements in technology in both healthcare and education. Many highly skilled healthcare professionals who understand, and who will progress, these technologies are an integral part of this movement (Gill, Gill & Young, 2013). In a fast-paced environment, many patients now tend to seek out an instant diagnosis, quick information or health treatment options from the internet before seeking professional advice (Ellis et al., 2013). The increasing advocacy for patient empowerment, primary prevention and effective self-management of one's own health has enthused many healthcare professionals and digital technology experts, encouraging them to further develop existing frameworks into a format for online, self-directed, patient education (Phillips et al., 2014; Yan, 2013). One absolute rationale for the development of digital education tools is the rapid evolution of digital technologies. To ensure both healthcare professionals and patients are ready, positive steps need to be taken to ensure that those intending to use or manage such systems are technologically literate (Gill, Gill & Young, 2013; Tom, 2014).

Discussion and critical thinking questions

7.1 What digital literacies do you think nursing students and other health-related students will need in the workplace of the future?

7.2 How are the technologies used for leisure now being used for study and in the workplace?

7.3 What are the likely consequences of future health professionals refusing to engage with new technologies? How is this likely to impact on patient care?

7.4 How can nursing students and other health-related students ensure patient privacy and confidentiality when using digital devices in the workplace?

7.5 How can social media be used effectively for disseminating a relevant message?

Learning extension

Think of the classrooms in which you have learnt. Has your learning experience always been perfect? Have the teaching techniques always catered to your learning style? Look back to the online learning resources detailed in the chapter. How do you think these compare with that classroom experience, and with live tutorials or lectures you have experienced? Can online learning cater to your learning style and those of others? Make a table of the pros and cons to how online education meets your learning needs. You will, of course, need to define your learning style.

Further reading

Gill, H.K., Gill, N. & Young, S.D. (2007). E-learning and professional development – never too old to learn. *British Journal of Nursing*, 16(17): 1084–8.

Roper, A. (2007). How students develop online learning skills. Successful online students share their secrets for getting the most from online classes, focusing on time management, active participation, and practice. *Educause Quarterly*, 1. Retrieved 20 November 2014 from <https://net.educause.edu/ir/library/pdf/EQM07110.pdf>.

References

Aleixo, C., Nunes, M. & Isaias, P. (2012). Usability and digital inclusion: Standards and guidelines. *International Journal of Public Administration*, 35(3): 221–39.

Aufderheide, P. (1992). *Media literacy: A report of the National Leadership Conference on Media Literacy*. Washington, DC: Aspen Institute.

Avila, J. & Pandya, J.Z. (2013). *Critical digital literacies as social praxis: Intersections and challenges*. New York: Peter Lang.

Ball, M., Smith, C. & Bakalar, R.S. (2006). Personal health records: Empowering consumers. *Journal of Healthcare Information Management*, 21(1): 76–86.

Beach, R., Bigelow, M., Dillon, D., Dockter, J., Galda, L. et al. (2009). *Annotated bibliography of research in the teaching of English*, vol. 44, pp. 210–41.

Bernat, J.L. (2013). Ethical and quality pitfalls in electronic health records. *Neurology*, 80(11): 1057–61.

Borgman, C.L. (2007). *Scholarship in the digital age: Information, infrastructure, and the internet*. Cambridge, MA: MIT Press.

Bowtell, L., Moloney, C., Kist, A.A., Parker, V., Maxwell, A. & Reedy, N. (2012). Enhancing nursing education with remote access laboratories. *International Journal of Online Engineering*, 8(2): 52–9.

Bozalek, V., Gachago, D., Alexander, L., Watters, K., Wood, D., Ivala, E. & Herrington, J. (2013). The use of emerging technologies for authentic learning: A South African study in higher education. *British Journal of Educational Technology*, 44(4), 629–38.

Brindley, P.G. & Reynolds, S.F. (2011). Improving verbal communication in critical care medicine. *Journal of Critical Care*, 26(2): 155–9.

Brown, R. (2012). Preliminary findings from a survey of student acceptance and use of e-textbooks in higher education. *Allied Academies International Conference: Proceedings of the Academy of Educational Leadership (AEL)*, 17(2): 1–5.

Chodos, D., Eleni, S., Boechler, P., King, S., Kuras, P., Carbonaro, M. & de Jong, E. (2010). Healthcare education with virtual-world simulations. Paper presented at the Software Engineering in Healthcare '10, Cape Town, South Africa. Retrieved 13 October 2014 from <http://dbonline.igroupnet.com/ACM. Ft/1810000/1809097/p89-chodos.pdf>.

Clark, L. (2009). Online skills fix aims to save HR staff jobs. *Personnel Today*, 4: 4.

Clifton, A. & Mann, C. (2011). Can YouTube enhance student nurse learning? *Nurse Education Today*, 31: 311–13.

Collier, A., Gray, B.J. & Ahn, M.J. (2011). Enablers and barriers to university and high technology SME partnerships. *Small Enterprise Research*, 18(1): 2–18.

Cui, G., Lockee, B. & Meng, C. (2013). Building modern online social presence: A review of social presence theory and its instructional design implications for future trends. *Education and Information Technologies*, 18(4): 661–85.

Dabbagh, N. & Kitsantas, A. (2011). Personal learning environments, social media, and self-regulated learning: A natural formula for connecting formal and informal learning. *Internet and Higher Education*, 15(1): 3–8.

Dabbagh, N. & Reo, R. (2011). Back to the future: Tracing the roots and learning affordances of social software. In M.J.W. Lee & C. McLoughlin (eds), *Web 2.0-based e-learning: Applying social informatics for tertiary teaching* (pp. 1–20). Hershey, PA: IGI Global.

Deepend (2014). *Australian mobile device ownership and home usage report 2014*. Sydney: Deepend.

Dudding, C.C. (2009). Digital videoconferencing: Applications across the disciplines. *Communication Disorders Quarterly*, 30(3): 178–82.

Duffy, M. (2012). Tablet technology for nursing. *American Journal of Nursing*, 112(9): 59–64.

Eisenberg, M.B. (2008). Information literacy: Essential skills for the information age. *DESIDOC Journal of Library & Information Technology*, 28(2): 39–47.

Ellis, L.A., Collin, P., Hurley, P.J., Davenport, T.A., Burns, J.M. & Hickie, I.B. (2013). Young men's attitudes and behaviour in relation to mental health and technology: Implications for the development of online mental health services. *BMC Psychiatry*, 13(1): 1–10.

Farley, H. (2011). Using multi-user virtual environments in tertiary teaching: Lessons learned through the UQ Religion Bazaar project. In C. Wankel (ed.), *Teaching arts and science with the new social media*. Bingley, UK: Emerald Group, pp. 211–37.

Gassert, C.A. (2000). Telehealth: A challenge to the regulation of multistate practice. *Policy, Politics & Nursing Practice*, 1(2): 85–92.

Giglia, E. (2011). Academic social networks: It's time to change the way we do research. *European Journal of Physical and Rehabilitation Medicine*, 47(2): 345–9.

Gill, H.K., Gill, N. & Young, S.D. (2013). Online technologies for health information and education: A literature review. *Journal of Consumer Health on the Internet*, 17(2): 139.

Govindan, M., Van Citters, A.D., Nelson, E.C., Kelly-Cummings, J. & Suresh, G. (2010). Automated detection of harm in healthcare with information technology: A systematic review. *Quality & Safety in Health Care*, 19(5): 1–11.

Greene, J.A., Yu, S.B. & Copeland, D.Z. (2014). Measuring critical components of digital literacy and their relationships with learning. *Computers & Education*, 76(5): 55–69.

Gyurko, C.C. & Ullmann, J. (2012). Using online technology to enhance educational mobility. *Online Journal of Nursing Informatics*, 16(1): 63–9.

Hamilton, E.C. & Friesen, N. (2013). Online education: A science and technology studies perspective. *Canadian Journal of Learning and Technology*, 39(2). Retrieved 20 January 2014 from <http://www.editlib.org/p/54417>.

Hargittai, E. & Litt, E. (2013). New strategies for employment? Internet skills and online privacy practices during people's job search. *IEEE Security & Privacy*, 11(3): 38–45.

Hazan, J.G. (2013). Stop being evil: A proposal for unbiased Google search. *Michigan Law Review*, 111(5): 789–820.

Herrington, J. & Parker, J. (2013). Emerging technologies as cognitive tools for authentic learning. *British Journal of Educational Technology*, 44(4): 607–15.

Hoerbst, A. & Ammenwerth, E. (2010). Electronic health records: A systematic review on quality requirements. *Methods of Information in Medicine*, 53(4): 235–7.

Horn, M.B. (2013). Digital roundup. *Education Next*, 13(4): 22–7.

Keengwe, J., Adjei-Boateng, E. & Diteeyont, W. (2013). Facilitating active social presence and meaningful interactions in online learning. *Education and Information Technologies*, 18(4): 597–607.

Kelland, J.H. (2011). Mixing personal and learning lives: How women mediate tensions when learning online. PhD thesis, University of Alberta. Retrieved 20 January 2014 from <http://www.editlib.org/p/122919>.

Koltay, M. (2011). The media and the literacies: Media literacy, information literacy, digital literacy. *Media, Culture & Society*, 33(2): 211–21.

Lasater, K., Johnson, E., Hodson-Carlton, K., Siktberg, L. & Sideras, S. (2012). A digital toolkit to implement and manage a multisite study. *Journal of Nursing Education*, 51(3): 127–32.

Lehnbom, E.C., Brien, J.E. & McLachlan, A.J. (2014). Knowledge and attitudes regarding the personally controlled electronic health record: An Australian national survey. *Internal Medicine Journal*, 44: 406–9.

Lukinbeal, C. (2014). Geographic media literacy. *Journal of Geography*, 113(2): 41–6.

Macdonald, J. (2004). Developing competent e-learners: The role of assessment. *Assessment & Evaluation in Higher Education*, 29(2): 215–26.

Martin, F., Parker, M. & Allred Oyarzun, B. (2013). A case study on the adoption and use of synchronous virtual classrooms. *Electronic Journal of e-Learning*, 11(2): 124–38.

McAllister, C. & Watkins, P. (2012). Increasing academic integrity in online classes by fostering the development of self-regulated learning skills. *Clearing House*, 85(3): 96–101.

McCallum, J., Ness, V. & Price, T. (2011). Exploring nursing students' decision-making skills whilst in a *Second Life* clinical simulation laboratory. *Nurse Education Today*, 31: 699–704.

McIntyre, M., McDonald, C. & Racine, L. (2013). A critical analysis of online nursing education: Balancing optimistic and cautionary perspectives. *Canadian Journal of Nursing Research (CJNR)*, 45(1): 36–53.

McLeod, S. & Barbara, A. (2005). Online technology in rural health: Supporting students to overcome the tyranny of distance. *Australian Journal of Rural Health*, 13(5): 276–81.

Miranda, L.C.M. & Lima, C.A.S. (2013). Technology substitution and innovation adoption: The cases of imaging and mobile communication markets. *Technological Forecasting and Social Change*, 80(6): 1179–93.

News, O. (2013). NZ smartphone ownership doubles in one year – study. *TVNZ*, 21 May. Retrieved 20 August 2014 from <http://tvnz.co.nz/technology-news/nz-smartphone-ownership-doubles-in-one-year-study-5443887>.

Nguyen, D.N., Zierler, B. & Nguyen, H.Q. (2011). A survey of nursing faculty needs for training in use of new technologies for education and practice. *Journal of Nursing Education*, 50(4): 181–9.

Pandey, S. & Pathak, M. (2014). A study on learners' perspective on learning management system in information technology industry. *International Journal of Information Technology & Computer Sciences Perspectives*, 3(2): 914–22.

Pearce, N., Weller, M., Scanlon, E. & Ashleigh, M. (2010). Digital scholarship considered: How new technologies could transform academic work. *e in education*, 16(1). Retrieved 20 January 2014 from <http://www.google.com.au/url?q= http://ineducation.ca/index.php/ineducation/article/download/44/509&sa= U&ei=Eh2_VJP2LejEmwWi1IHYCA&ved=0CBQQFjAA&usg= AFQjCNGx1r6txfYBrgbSvm3iDG5v6hDLMQ>.

Peters, M.A. (2004). Editorial: E-learning machines. *E-Learning*, 1(1): 1–8.

Phillips, J.L., Heneka, N., Hickman, L., Lam, L. & Shaw, T. (2014). Impact of a novel online learning module on specialist palliative care nurses' pain assessment competencies and patients' reports of pain: Results from a quasi-experimental pilot study. *Palliative Medicine*, 28(6): 521–9.

Reynolds, D.W., Murray, C.M. & Germany, R.E. (2008). Device therapy for remote patient therapy. In I. Gussack, C. Antzelevitch, A.A.M. Wilde, P.A. Friedman, M.J. Ackerman & W.-K. Shen (eds), *Electrical diseases of the heart: Genetics, mechanisms, treatment, prevention*. London: Springer-Verlag, pp. 809–25.

Rockinson-Szapkiw, A.J., Courduff, J., Carter, K. & Bennett, D. (2013). Electronic versus traditional print textbooks: A comparison study on the influence of university students' learning. *Computers & Education*, 63: 259–66.

Roper, A.R. (2007). How students develop online learning skills. *EDUCAUSE Quarterly*, 30(1): 62–5.

Rowland, L., Canning, N., Faulhaber, D., Lingle, W. & Redgrave, A. (2014). A multiliteracies approach to materials analysis. *Language, Culture and Curriculum*, 27(2): 136–50.

Santos, C., Brogueira, G. & Bernardino, C. (2014). Social networks with BuddyPress. Paper presented at the Proceedings of the International Conference on Information Systems and Design of Communication, Lisbon, Portugal.

Sawyer, E.A. & Howard, C. (2007). Online learning program strategic planning and execution: Considering goals, benefits, problems and communities of practice. *Journal of College Teaching & Learning*, 4(8): 99–112.

Shen, D., Cho, M.-H., Tsai, C.-L. & Marra, R. (2013). Unpacking online learning experiences: Online learning self-efficacy and learning satisfaction. *The Internet and Higher Education*, 19(3–4): 10–17.

Sinha, P. & Poggio, T. (1996). Role of learning in three-dimensional form perception. *Nature*, 384(6608): 460–3.

Smith, C. (2014). New picture-sharing app for doctors, medical students raises privacy concerns, *ABC News*, 14 April. Retrieved 20 June 2014 from <http://www.abc.net.au/news/2014-04-14/picture-sharing-app-for-doctors-raises-privacy-concerns/5389226>.

Stiftung, B. (2009). Patient-centred electronic health records. *Health Policy Monitor*. Auckland: University of Auckland.

Sur, E., Ünal, E. & İşeri, K. (2014). Primary school second grade teachers' and students' opinions on media literacy. *Creencias sobre alfabetización mediática en profesores y estudiantes de Educación Primaria*, 21(42): 119–27.

Tan, L. & Guo, L. (2014). Multiliteracies in an outcome-driven curriculum: Where is its fit? *Asia-Pacific Education Researcher*, 23(1): 29–36.

Taras, V.A.S., Caprar, D.V., Rottig, D., Sarala, R.M., Zakaria, N. et al. (2013). A global classroom? Evaluating the effectiveness of global virtual collaboration as a teaching tool in management education. *Academy of Management Learning & Education*, 12(3): 414–35.

Thompson, L.F. & Lynch, B.J. (2003). Web-based instruction: Who is inclined to resist it and why? *Journal of Educational Computing Research*, 29(3): 375–85.

Tom, P.-A. (2014). The technology of teaching. *American School & University*, 86(7): 16–21.

Warschauer, M. (2001). Online communication. In R. Carter & D. Nunan (eds), *The Cambridge guide to teaching English to speakers of other languages*. Cambridge: Cambridge University Press, pp. 207–12.

Welsh, J. (2012). Safeguarding people who are at risk of abuse. *Emergency Nurse*, 20(5): 14–17.

Wetterneck, T.B., Skibinski, K.A., Roberts, T.L., Kleppin, S.M., Schroeder, M.E. et al. (2006). Using failure mode and effects analysis to plan implementation of smart IV pump technology. *American Journal of Health-System Pharmacy*, 63(16): 1528–38.

Wong, Y.C., Fung, J.Y.C., Law, C.K., Lam, J.C.Y. & Lee, V.W.P. (2009). Tackling the digital divide. *The British Journal of Social Work*, 39(4): 754–67.

Wright, D. (2013). Communication and cultural change in university technology transfer. *Journal of Technical Writing & Communication*, 43(1): 79–101.

Yan, L. (2013). The value of social media for patients: Social supports, networking, and learning in online healthcare communities. PhD thesis, University of Southern Queensland. Retrieved 12 November 2014 from <http://ezproxy.usq.edu.au/login?url=http://search.ebscohost.com/login. aspx?direct=true&db=psyh&AN=2013–99151–060&site=ehost-live>.

8

Professional skills for nurses and other health professionals

CONTEXTS AND CAPABILITY OF PRACTICE

Cheryl Perrin, David Stanley and Melissa Taylor

Learning objectives

- Develop an understanding of the structure and functions of healthcare organisations.

- Assess the impact of organisational structure and culture on contexts of practice.

- Appreciate the importance of professional communication, team membership and emotional intelligence on practice capability.

- Develop an understanding of leadership and management in healthcare.

- Identify the importance of effective clinical leadership for practice capability.

- Recognise and understand the links between leadership, scope of practice, quality initiatives and evidence-informed practice.

Key terms

- Clinical leadership

- Congruent leadership

- Emotional intelligence

- Evidence informed practice (EIP)

- Healthcare team

- Leadership

- Management

- Organisation

- Organisational culture

- Professional communication

- Quality initiatives

Introduction

The dynamic and evolving healthcare systems of the twenty-first century require healthcare professionals to be cognisant of the various influences on their capabilities and contexts of practice. This chapter provides insights into some of these influences to assist you to develop an understanding of how the 'big-picture' influences can shape the practice settings or practice contexts in which you work on a day-to-day basis. Initially, the structure and function of organisations and their organisational cultures will be discussed, along with the important components of professional communication, being part of an effective team and the influence of **emotional intelligence** on practice capability. It is also important to know and understand the application of the terms **leadership** and **management** when applied in a healthcare setting, including the significance of appreciating the concept of clinical leadership, which forms an important link to a health professional's scope of practice and their capacity to influence practice and patient outcomes. These threads continue throughout the chapter, with the linking of leadership, scope of practice, quality initiatives and **evidence-informed practice (EIP)**.

emotional intelligence: the emotional and social characteristics, skills and enablers that determine how we perceive and express ourselves, understand and relate to others, and cope with daily living

leadership: undertaken or carried out by people who try to unify people around values and then construct the social world for others around those values

management: the process of leading and directing all or part of an organisation through the deployment and manipulation of resources

evidence-informed practice (EIP): ensuring health practice is guided by the best research and information available

Contexts of practice

What do we actually mean when we talk about a practice context? In this chapter, we are referring to your area of healthcare or practice setting. As you know, this can mean almost anywhere there are healthcare professionals and consumers of care. Healthcare contexts are complex environments, and they have multiple components that impact on their structure, functions and the ability of those within them to provide care. The local community, the local environment, and the political and economic circumstances all affect practice contexts, which in turn influence the leadership, management, capacity and capability of healthcare employees. This chapter focuses on some of the components that impact on contexts of practice.

Understanding healthcare organisational structures

All of us belong to several different **organisations**. We might be a member of a sporting organisation, a professional organisation and/or a social organisation. We tend not to think consciously about their description as an organisation because we see them as specific components of our lives that allow us to reach our goals by following rules and processes set with a group of like-minded people. These organisations are simply a part of our day-to-day lives. Each organisation with which we interact – whether it is large or small – influences varying aspects of our lives.

organisation: a collection of individuals brought together in a particular environment to achieve a set of pre-determined objectives

Organisations impact on the ways in which communities and groups within communities operate. They influence the way policies and standards are defined, monitored and enacted, the authority and communication pathways used, and how goods and services such as healthcare are provided by governments and other agencies. Mancini (2015a) notes that external factors such as economics, social structures and demographics are major interactive components that influence the actual structure, mission statement and philosophy of the organisation. These internal and external elements also influence the level of satisfaction of employees who work within the organisation, the people who may reside within an organisation such as a residential care facility, and those in the surrounding communities who access the resources provided by the organisation, such as healthcare.

We understand the impact of these elements when we hear, see and read about changes in healthcare delivery systems that are the result of the prevailing politico-economic and social climate in the country. Flowing on from these are changes to nursing roles and how care is provided – elements that will continue to change as organisations respond to both internal and external influences. While Hein's (1998) description of an organisation as a 'living organism with interactive parts' was written some years ago, it remains a good analogy today.

All organisations have a formal structure, which determines the roles of the individuals within the organisation, how the power and decision-making are delegated, how resources are allocated and the communication pathways within the organisation. The major organisational structures identified in the literature include the tall or bureaucratic organisation, the functional structure, the flat or decentralised organisation and the matrix structure (Ellis & Hartley, 2009; Mancini, 2015b). Mancini (2015b) writes that bureaucracies historically have been described in a negative fashion as a tall structure with the decision-making flowing from the top down to the workers, with clear lines of labour and control. The traditional bureaucratic structure keeps control at the top, giving little or no autonomy to the workers at the lower levels. The modern versions may possess some of these characteristics, but they often delegate autonomy and authority to some workers so the organisation can deliver its services and meet its goals, mission and philosophy more effectively. If you look at large healthcare organisations, you will see elements of a bureaucracy with aspects of a functional structure evident. Functional structures are very common in healthcare organisations. According to Mancini (2015b), the functional structure enables specialities to be housed within departments that offer similar services, with the department manager or supervisor reporting to a head of a major over-arching area. Both of these types of structure have clearly defined rules of reporting and lines of authority. Alternatively, the flat or decentralised organisation has less rigidity and more flexibility, as the management structure has been 'flattened' with the removal of a layer of management (Grohar-Murray & Langan, 2011). Matrix structures, on the other hand, are an integrated matrix of teams within a functional, bureaucratic structure that enables effective communication and consultation between **healthcare teams** in order to handle the diverse range of problems and specialities that can be found in a healthcare system (Grohar-Murray & Langan, 2011).

> **healthcare team:** a group of people with common health goals and objectives, who work together to meet them

What do these structure look like? Figure 8.1 gives a visual representation of how an organisation chart might look, showing the formal relationships and lines of communication and reporting within that particular organisation.

Create an organisational chart for an organisation with which you are familiar. It might be the sports club to which you belong or an organisation where you have been employed. Fill in the lines of control and communication, and include specialist areas where appropriate. If it is a large, complex organisation, you might concentrate on a department or section and draw how it would fit into the bigger picture. When you have completed the chart, write out your responses to the following questions, explaining (with references to relevant literature) whether this structure enables the organisation to deliver its goals effectively:

> Does the organisation have a bureaucratic, flat, functional or matrix structure?
> Are there open communication channels?
> How does the chain of command operate?

LEARNING ACTIVITY

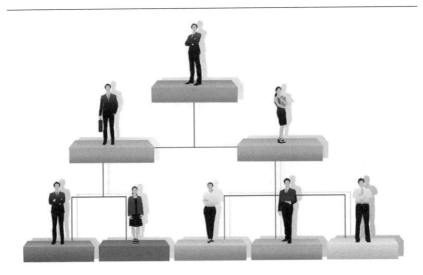

FIGURE 8.1 *Illustration of an organisational chart*

> What is the organisational mission statement?
> Does the organisational structure enable the achievement of the mission statement?
> What changes could be made to provide a better fit between the organisational structure and the mission statement?

Informal organisational structures

Now you have an understanding of formal organisational structures and the concepts of the chain of command, power and control, and lines of communication, it is time to look at the informal structures that exist within organisations. These do not show up on the formal organisational chart, yet they have a considerable impact on the practice context of employees, as this is where the majority of the organisation's communication takes place (Ellis & Hartley, 2009). Ellis and Hartley (2009) note that the informal structure is as essential to the functioning of the organisation as the formal structure. It provides the social and communication infrastructure that assists employees to feel happy at work, and to achieve their goals through cooperation and communication. Hein's (1998) seminal work on informal organisational structures takes a different viewpoint, discussing the idea that the informal structures will often give a more accurate indication of the state of the formal structure – particularly if there is general dissatisfaction with the work environment. As healthcare workers continue to deal with rapidly changing practice contexts, role challenges and increasing work-related stressors, there is a growing awareness of the need to look more closely at the impact – both positive and negative – of informal organisational structures.

Organisational culture

Organisational culture is not always an easy concept to understand. According to Mancini (2015a), the culture of an organisation is interlinked with the values and beliefs, or norms and traditions, of the organisation, and includes both the formal and informal structure and functions. For example, the formal organisational culture can be seen in the written documents such as the organisation's mission, vision and philosophy statements, policies and procedures, and organisational position descriptions, while the informal culture is found in the daily experiences of employees. Do employees feel comfortable that what is written really reflects how staff and patients are treated, or is there dissonance between the two (Mancini, 2015a)? Jones and Bennett (2012) cite French and Bell's (1990) iceberg model of organisational climate, noting that the formal or tangible components are visible while the intangibile components – such as values, attitudes, perceptions, routines and stories around the everyday activities of the organisation – are hidden. These authors also note that the culture of an organisation will be influenced by the structure, and by the levels of power and control within and between employee groups.

> **organisational culture:** reflects the norms or traditions of the organisation and is exemplified by behaviours that illustrate values and beliefs

Teams in healthcare

Nurses working each day within the healthcare sector need to have a good understanding of the organisational culture with which their work is conducted. Knowing how to manage different staff perceptions, routines and the culture within healthcare work is important, as it is these intangible concepts that shape the culture and perceptions of individuals and ultimately affect how work is conducted and the way communication occurs in teams (MacKian & Simons, 2013). Within healthcare, team approaches to care delivery are common, so the ability to work with and understand the people within health teams is important. While a team will always be constructed of multiple different personalities, gender differences, cultural and social differences, what matters is how each of these differences is negotiated, accepted and tolerated, and establishing a consensus within the team to ensure the common aim of quality care delivery is achieved.

Power and team influence

Many variables have an impact on the success of teams. One critical key to success is effective communication within and between individual team members. In a clinical setting, there are individuals who make things happen through indirect power and influence. Such individuals are present in all workplaces: they are people who make those things that impact on the level and quality of care at the bedside happen. They have the power to affect other people's thinking and often change the way work is done (Stanley, 2011). These individuals can be categorised as those who are willing to share knowledge, are liked by colleagues for their professional capability, have the capacity to maintain a cohesive team, and are able to communicate well with everyone at both a clinical ward level or a management level.

Professional communication

Professional communication between healthcare professionals and the patients/clients within the health service is critical. What is said and what is not said often shape the perceptions of the care provided. This includes the trust and rapport of the healthcare providers and the individuals' approach and attitude towards their professional communication. For example, the communication might be from nurse to nurse (intra-professional) or between different members of the healthcare team, such as doctors, pharmacists, physiotherapists and nurses (inter-professional) (see Chapter 2). The leader of a healthcare team allocates care according to the clinical demands of the day. For example, the registered nurse will use their decision-making ability in line with clinical needs, staff relations and organisational capacity.

professional communication: a process by which information, perception and understanding are transmitted from person to person

Practice statements relating to leadership and communication are well documented in the nursing literature and the professional nursing codes of ethics and standards of professional practice in Australia; these are integral to the role of the registered nurse (Acree, 2006; Avolio & Bass, 1999; Dignam et al., 2012; NMBA, 2006). The *National Competency Standards for the Registered Nurse*

(NMBA, 2006) identify the characteristics of leadership as being inherent within the practice of a registered nurse. For this reason, all registered nurses play a role in leadership in the clinical environment, irrespective of their level of expertise. This is inclusive of care planning, delivery, evaluation, referral and consultation with members of the multidisciplinary team. The ways in which this is communicated and conveyed effectively within the team are essential to patient care, standards of practice, and personal and professional development (Anderson & Helms, 2000; MacKian & Simons, 2013; Stanley, 2006a; Thompson, 2012).

Vertical and horizontal communication

To communicate successfully in teams, nurses must be able to communicate both horizontally and vertically within the team.

Horizontal communication

Horizontal communication refers to communication with other members of the team, each of whom forms a direct part of the team. For example, a typical team on a morning shift within a busy 36-bed medical ward could include one clinical nurse, three registered nurses, two enrolled nurses and two personal care workers. The handover is provided to the staff and a work allocation of patients is distributed among the group. This team nursing approach to care is common, and both verbal and written communication is essential to the coordination of care and operational management (Anderson & Helms, 2000; Bokhour, 2006). Nurses are required to work cooperatively with each individual, interacting effectively, providing feedback, accepting and being involved in critical discussions and exhibiting the capacity to self-reflect (Bokhour, 2006; Ortega et al., 2013).

Throughout the shift on the medical ward, many tasks are conducted that are based on patient needs, activities of daily living, diagnosis and treatment plans, medical and healthcare team 'rounds' and resultant care-planning decisions in a nursing and medical and healthcare team context. This horizontal primary communication is directly related to care provided, and is aimed at quality patient outcomes. Communication tools like ISOBAR or ISBAR provide health professionals with structured communication pathways to communicate care decisions (ACSQHC, 2011) (see Chapter 2).

Vertical communication

Vertical communication within the healthcare team is an example of two-way communication. It is through vertical communication that healthcare management provides information to employees and receives information from staff about corporate progress or concerns within an organisation. This type of communication includes both upward and downward communication, and the conveying of information occurs through established channels or communication portals (MacKian & Simons, 2013).

Effective team communication and the capability to lead within a team are complex and multifaceted qualities. There is no 'normal' routine; however, the way we send and receive messages and what is done with the content are critical. This process affects the leadership styles, the power of individuals and the trust and respect that develop in teams, where communication and feedback play a pivotal role.

Emotional intelligence in nursing

The concept of emotional intelligence (EI) is essential in a clinical team, as it ensures effective team interaction and productivity, and is imperative for effective coordination of the team. Emotional intelligence can be identified in the power or drive shown by informal leaders in motivating the team towards collective action, facilitating or mentoring supportive relationships and inspiring a transformational influence within the team (MacKian & Simons, 2013; McCloskey et al., 1996). Individuals with emotional intelligence have the skills necessary to both manage and lead a team proactively; they possess both the skill and ability to inspire others to achieve common goals (MacKian & Simons, 2013; McQueen, 2004).

To assist nurses to determine how to use concepts of emotional intelligence within their practice, Goleman's (1998) model of emotional intelligence is further elaborated upon below. The model has five elements:

1 *Self-awareness.* This means having a deeper understanding of personal emotions, including strengths and weaknesses; possessing an honest demeanour and being able to self-reflect on events and situations.

2 *Self-regulation.* This is the ability to be able to effectively manage internal stressors in a calm and non-confronting way when facing a challenging or difficult situation. The art of self-regulation is the ability to be able to remain calm, think through decisions and communicate calmly and responsibly; it is not about demanding or acting on impulsive decisions.

3 *Motivation.* Motivated leaders understand goals and dreams, and have developed skills of self-reflection. Their work is constructed around engaging staff to achieve a shared vision. For example, this could be seen through inspiring staff and gaining their commitment to a project.

4 *Empathy.* To be empathetic within the healthcare setting is to be aware of other people's feelings, needs and concerns. This is particularly vital with regard to peer support and awareness of colleagues who work in our teams; a leader needs to have the ability to manage their emotions and maintain a level of self-control and calm.

5 *Social skills.* This is also inclusive of a level of empathy with others – that is, the ability to listen to and comprehend other people's perspectives and to act in the best interests of staff and the organisation.

Many of these elements are core concepts in this book.

Clinical capability

Clinical capability is far greater than having the ability to perform a role. In determining the capability of a team, it is important to understand how a team carries out daily care provisions within a ward or department, and how effective communication and delegation of care occur within the team. Delegation can be summarised as entrusting a task or responsibility to another – typically someone less senior than you (McCloskey et al., 1996). It is *not* ordering or telling someone to do something; however, it could be described as asking someone to do something – in a non-threatening and engaging way.

Delegation assigns responsibility from one member of the team to another. It is imperative that instructions relating to the task being delegated are clear and concise, thus making it clear that the person is now responsible for the outcome. This responsibility instils a sense of authority within the individual who is now responsible for accomplishing the task. It is vital to this success that the delegate now has, or is explicitly given, the power to accomplish the task.

Feedback and accountability go hand in hand. Delegation must ensure that staff to whom a task/responsibility is delegated :

- have the skills to perform the task
- accept responsibility for performing the task
- have the authority to perform the task within their registration, position description and organisational policy or procedure.

The *National Competency Standards for the Registered Nurse* (NMBA, 2006) identify circumstances where delegation of a specific duty is not appropriate, or remains outside the scope of practice of a particular practitioner within the team. It is not appropriate for a registered nurse to delegate patient care planning, patient assessments, collaboration of care, education and evaluation of clients, or any primary teaching responsibilities to an enrolled nurse or personal care worker/assistant in nursing.

It is often difficult to acknowledge the need to effectively delegate care when working within healthcare teams, particularly in nursing teams. It is important to be able to communicate within teams, and to have the inspiration and motivation to succeed. A resistance to delegation can create a barrier within nurses who feel a need to complete all caring for the patients within their allocation. These barriers can add to elements of poor communication and include the notion that to delegate caring would take too long to explain to others or create a team perception that 'the staff with whom I work wouldn't like me'. Often our perceptions of what others in the team would think create barriers within nursing teams, preventing us from effectively delegating and communicating care and ultimately adding to power imbalances and miscommunications (see Chapters 2 and 3).

Effective delegation has five steps:

1 Identify the key task.
2 Delegate each task appropriately.
3 Explain each task to the team/team member.
4 Develop a plan (how will it be accomplished and by when?).
5 Monitor progress but don't micro-manage the task.

Using these steps within a healthcare team can help to provide a conducive environment for staff and patients to create quality outcomes. If the process is used correctly, an environment is created that is more productive, fosters creativity and opportunity, focuses on communication and ensures greater team and individual accountability. Delegation and team communication are not as easy as they sound. Managing complex personalities, feeling comfortable with personal and inter-professional communication and being comfortable with personal and professional clinical decision-making are just some of the key ingredients for success.

Think about the area in which you currently work (within healthcare or another industry). Respond to the following in relation to your workplace:

1 Identify your accountability as a student in the clinical area.
2 Are you able to delegate tasks or responsibilities to other nursing staff?
3 Explain your answer to Question 2.

Ben's story

Ben has been working on a busy surgical unit since completing his graduate program nine months ago. He thoroughly enjoys the work on the ward; however, he has had problems getting on with some of the staff. The new roster has just been released and Ben is keen to see whether he has a particular weekend off as he is hoping to spend the weekend with his friends. On scanning the roster, Ben notices that he is rostered for an early shift on the Saturday of the weekend days off that he had requested. He feels uncomfortable about asking another staff member to swap with him. At handover, he finds he is working the evening with two senior registered nurses with whom he has communication challenges.

Critical reflection

1   What key concerns can you identify in Ben's professional communication challenges?

2   What communication strategies could Ben use to improve his inter-personal communication skills?

Ben has been allocated the role of 'team leader' within his section, and has been teamed with a casual enrolled nurse and another registered nurse. Ben describes this registered nurse as always busy and not easy to approach for assistance. Consequently, Ben feels he has to just get on with his workload allocation. The shift progresses and Ben begins with an assessment of his patients. He has 12 patients. Five are post-operative, two are new admissions for surgery, two patients are ready for discharge and require discharge planning, and three are awaiting surgical review.

The enrolled nurse asks Ben how he would like the work divided. The registered nurse working with Ben announces that they are heading for a tea break before starting.

Critical reflection

>>   Consider the following question in relation to Ben's story. What is a team and why do teams matter?

>>   Using the five elements of Goleman's (1998) model of emotional intelligence, describe how you would address each element in the table below:

ELEMENT	ACTION
Self-awareness	
Self-regulation	
Motivation	
Empathy	
Social skills	

What are leadership and management in healthcare?

Leadership and management are essentially skill sets and, like any other skills to which health professionals aspire, they need to be understood and practised for them to be refined and employed effectively. Commonly, the terms 'leader' and 'manager' are also used to describe a person's position, job title or career level, with the implication that the position holder will embody these skills. However, nurses and other health professionals 'manage' even without the title (management of workloads, patient care, equipment and a range of delegated duties). They often lead informally as part of a team, in a multi-professional group, or because patients look to them for direction, care and guidance. Therefore, in healthcare, it is vital to understand leadership and management so these skill sets can be grasped and applied, like any other clinical or technical skill and knowledge held by nurses and health professionals (Jones & Bennett, 2012; Stanley, 2011).

Leadership

There are many definitions of leadership, and over the years these have continued to be refined. Key aspects of past definitions include the premise that to be a leader one needs followers, even if the leader is not aware of them (Kean et al., 2011); that leadership is related to an 'influence relationship' (Jones & Bennett, 2012, p. 2); that leadership focuses on change and new directions or initiative, innovation and new outcomes (sometimes linked to vision) (Bennis & Nanus, 1985; Burns, 1978); and that the leader holds true to their values and beliefs, and has a strong sense of self-belief (Clark, 2008; Stanley, 2011). Indeed, Zaleznik (1977) believes a leader's goals arise out of a personal or passionate desire to infuse meaning into the world. Leaders are therefore about people and the meaning of actions for them. They ask the 'Why not?' question and, according to Bennis and Nanus (1985), 'do the right thing', while managers 'do things right'. Kotter (1990) understands that leadership is rooted in the maxim that the more change there is, the more leadership is required. Central to an understanding of leadership is the recognition that leadership is about coping with change. Part of the reason why leadership (particularly in the health services) has become such an issue is that the more change there is, the greater is the demand for more leadership.

It is a common misconception that leaders hold apex or top-level positions in an organisation, department or ward. The reality is that leaders exist at all levels of an organisation (Jones & Bennett, 2012; Stanley, 2011), and the value of understanding a wider definition of leadership is that it points to the ability of anyone who is prepared to do the right thing, has self-belief and is prepared to exercise their influence by staying true to their values and beliefs in order to be seen as a leader. In this light, Warren (2005) sees leaders as being at the 'heart of an organisation', with leadership acting as a relationship between the leader and the led that can energise the organisation.

Management

Managers can certainly be leaders; however, Warren (2005) states that management consists of three things: analysis, problem-solving and planning. It is proposed that management may be seen as being more about the business and less about the people, with people being viewed only as important for getting the job done. Kotter (1990) understands management to be about coping with complexity. It has evolved because, without good management, large organisations and complex enterprises tend to become chaotic. Good managers bring order and consistency to key dimensions like quality and profitability. Management is therefore about consistency and stability (Kotter, 1990).

The difference between leadership and management in healthcare

Kotter (1990) sees a distinction between a leader and a manager. Leaders align people, set direction, motivate, inspire, employ credibility and cope with change. Managers plan and budget, set goals and targets, organise and sort staffing, control, problem-solve and cope with complexity. Management needs to be exercised in any business or organisation; leadership is an essential part of a business or organisation if that business or organisation is to grow, change and develop. Both leadership and management are essential for the success of an organisation or business, and while they are not the same thing, they do complement each other (Dignam et al., 2012; Long, 2011). The health services are very complex, and could not function without effective management. Their potential to grow and respond to new medical and healthcare advances is only possible with the flashes of creativity and vision that insightful leaders bring, and the application of these through the leaders' values and beliefs. Long's (2011) suggestion is that the separation of management and leadership could be harmful or dangerous may ring true from an organisational perspective. From a clinical standpoint, differences in the focus and motivation of leadership and management can potentially lead to conflict, confusion, poor-quality healthcare and diminished clinical and managerial effectiveness (Stanley, 2006a).

Clinical leadership and practice capability

While 'leadership' and 'nursing leadership', or 'healthcare leadership', are terms that have been evident in nursing and health industry literature for many decades, **clinical leadership** is a relatively new term that remains ill-defined (Mannix, Wilkes & Daly, 2013). Many authors, researchers and clinicians have contributed to our understanding of clinical leadership. Peach (1995) and Lett (2002) (both from an Australian perspective) and the American authors Dean-Barr (1998), McCormack and Hopkins (1995) and Rocchiccioli and Tilbury (1998) have contributed to the dialogue. Berwick (1994), Wyatt (1995) and Schneider (1999) (from a medical and pharmacological standpoint) have also added to the discussion. Swanwick and McKimm (2011) have offered considerable text on this topic. Harper (1995) offered the earliest nursing definition, with others such as Cook (2001a, 2001b) (from the United Kingdom) also helping to build the body of knowledge on the topic.

> **clinical leadership:**
> putting clinicians at the heart of shaping and running clinical services to deliver excellent outcomes for patients and populations as a core part of clinicians' professional identity

Summarising all their contributions offers a view that clinical leaders can be seen as:

- having clinical expertise
- being an expert nurse or expert in their field
- being directly involved in clinical care
- possessing excellent interpersonal skills, or being able to influence others
- being approachable and effective communicators
- acting as role models and motivators
- being focused on quality patient care, and better health and healthcare

- improving care and maintaining high standards so that excellent outcomes for patients and populations are delivered
- being empowered, empowering others and transforming services because they remain focused on their values and beliefs
- promoting the values of their profession or organisation and seeing these qualities as a core part of a clinician's professional identity.

Interestingly, the reality was seldom linked directly to the definitions offered, with clinical leaders more likely to be recognised and followed because they matched their values and beliefs with their actions in clinical practice (Stanley 2006b, 2008, 2011, 2014). Stanton, Lemer and Mountford (2010, p. 5) offer the view that anyone who is in a clinical role and who exercises leadership is a clinical leader. They also suggest that a clinical leader's role is to 'empower clinicians to have the confidence and capability to continually improve healthcare on both the small and the large scale'. The UK Department of Health (2007, p. 49) defines the role of clinical leaders:

> To motivate, to inspire, to promote the values of the NHS, to empower and create a consistent focus on the needs of patients being served. Leadership is necessary not just to maintain high standards of care, but to transform services to achieve even higher levels of excellence.

These definitions capture the idea that clinical leaders are in non-hierarchical or informal positions, and are directly involved in enhancing clinical care by influencing others (Clark, 2008; Cook, 2001a; Downey, Parslow & Smart, 2011). Cook and Holt (2000) support this perspective, suggesting that clinical leaders are involved in clinical care, have a relationship with quality patient care and are able to influence others. This implies that clinical leaders may not need to be in positions of power, or hold significant hierarchical positions, to lead in the clinical arena. As well, they state that clinical leaders must be good communicators, and that they need effective team-building skills and respect for others.

The attributes of clinical leaders

Cook (2001a, p. 33) attempted to identify the attributes of effective clinical leaders by focusing not on nurses at the 'hierarchical apex of the organisation ... but on those nurses that directly deliver nursing care'. Cook's study focused on nurses who were not deemed to be in conventional nursing leadership positions, but who displayed many of the attributes of highly effective leaders. Although based on only a limited study, this research identified 'typologies' associated with clinical leaders, including discoverers, valuers, enablers, shapers and modifiers. Significantly, having a vision, developing a vision or articulating a vision were not central themes in Cook's clinical leadership research.

Hurley and Hutchinson (2013) and Mannix, Wilkes and Daly (2013) have undertaken reviews of Australian literature on leadership and clinical leadership respectively. Each study concluded that only limited research studies exist, and that challenges remain for researchers looking at this topic. However, research by Stanley (2014) over a number of years, with a number of health professional groups in different countries, identified the following attributes as constantly present in clinical leaders in the health services: being approachable, clinically competent, motivated, supportive, inspiring confidence, a role model for others, a mentor, an effective communicator, visible in practice and acting in concert with their personal values and beliefs. Cook's (2001a) study identified similar results, with clinical leaders also being recognised for their ability to support others, motivate and empower, make decisions, and value both themselves and others. Berwick (1994) and Schneider (1999), in relation to clinical leadership from a medical and pharmacological perspective, also saw clinical expertise as central to the characteristics of a clinical leader. Clinical leaders were therefore recognisable because they possessed a set of knowledge that was specific to their clinical field. While this knowledge base may have extended into a broad range of topics or areas, clinical leaders were often recognisable because they had knowledge of and could undertake the activities central to their field of practice. These attributes, combined with effective communication skills, both in terms of listening to and engaging with others and being open, approachable and visible in the clinical area, were central in order for clinical leaders to be seen as role models for professional or clinical practice.

Practice capacity and capability

Clinical leaders can be found in all areas of care. They may not be the manager or even the most senior healthcare professional in the clinical area, but they are represented by clinicians who are visible in practice and identified by their values and beliefs about care (Cook, 2001b; Downey, Parslow & Smart, 2011; Stanley, 2014). They could be a student nurse, a nursing assistant, a newly registered nurse, a very experienced nurse or indeed any other member of the healthcare team. As clinical leaders can be at any level, they have the capacity to influence practice across the spectrum of interventions. This is a key aspect of understanding clinical leadership, because it implies that any clinician can influence and lead innovation or change practice that has the potential to benefit and improve care for patients or clients (Stanley, 2011).

Linking clinical leadership to scope of practice, quality initiatives and evidence-informed practice

Debora's story (see the Case study) offers a useful example of the application of clinical leadership to practice. As part of their scope of practice requirements, all registered nurses must be accountable for their practice, and protect individuals and groups within ethical and legal guidelines. As well, registered nurses are required to employ evidence-based practice, reflect on practice and base their practice on evidence-based interventions (see Chapter 9). In addition, they should work collaboratively and build professional relationships (NMBA, 2006).

Debora's story: A FAST HUG

Case study

Debora was a newly qualified registered nurse working in an intensive care unit (ICU). After starting work in the unit, she realised that each nurse undertook their care and assessments responsibilities differently, and that this made it difficult for her to learn what assessments and care should be provided as a minimum with each ICU patient. Debora realised that this resulted in the provision of inconsistent care across the unit. Reading a nursing journal one day, she came across an article that described the mnemonic FAST HUG, which consisted of a care checklist and suggested interventions for dealing with critically ill patients. The FAST

HUG mnemonic means: **F**eeding, **A**nalgesia, **S**edation, **T**hromboembolic prophylaxis, **H**ead-of-bed elevation, stress **U**lcer prevention and **G**lucose control. Recognising the potential benefits of this system, she raised the introduction of a FAST HUG via a trial in the ICU. After some initial reluctance, a number of staff agreed that it had the potential to offer more consistent care and, with the support of the unit manager, a trial was arranged and undertaken. After six months and a number of hurdles that needed to be overcome, the trial was evaluated as a success, and the FAST HUG system of assessment and intervention management was introduced permanently into the ICU.

Debora demonstrated initiative as a clinical leader, despite her limited clinical experience in ICU or as a registered nurse. She was able to reflect upon her practice and that of her colleagues. She identified another approach to care, leading to a proposal to modify the clinical practice in the ICU in a way that enhanced patient care and improved quality care outcomes.

This example shows that effective clinical leaders work within their professional standards to seek out and develop innovations that impact positively on patient/client care and lead to better healthcare outcomes. Central to the capacity to do this well is the use of clear and effective communication, excellent negotiation and networking skills, and the ability to work collaboratively, inclusively and respectfully. All these skills point to the qualities and attributes of effective clinical leaders, working towards evidence informed practice and employing **congruent leadership** (Stanley, 2008, 2011). Clinical leaders apply their values and beliefs about quality patient care by following up on what they believe to be in the best interests of the health service, their clinical area and the patients or clients it supports.

congruent leadership: when a leader establishes a match (or congruence) between their values and beliefs and their actions

> › Describe how leadership and management complement one another.
> › Think about someone to whom you have looked up as a leader in clinical practice. What leadership attributes did they demonstrate?

Summary

The formal and informal elements of healthcare agencies and organisations affect the practice contexts, capacity and capability of healthcare professionals. They are indicators of the congruence (or lack of it) between the values and mission of an organisation, and the staff perceptions and feelings about the organisation. Understanding the culture of an organisation will assist you to reflect on your role in the team, and the extent to which your values and goals align with those of the organisation. Teams and team-building, professional communication and emotional intelligence are also profound influences on how healthcare workers are able to function within organisations. Leadership is about dealing with and supporting change innovations, while management is about stability, consistency and dealing with large, chaotic organisations. While leadership and management are not the same, they may complement each other so that organisations, wards and departments can be managed well and led effectively in order to deal with future change and responses to client needs. Clinical leaders are the clinical experts directly involved in providing clinical care. They are the approachable role models of congruent leadership who communicate and inspire others with actions that embody their values and beliefs about care. This clinical leadership is linked to the appropriate applica-tion of a nurse's scope of practice by the integration of **quality initiatives** and the application of evidence-informed practice to improve care standards and provide the best care possible for recipients.

quality initiatives: actions taken within the healthcare system that strive to provide safe, high-quality healthcare, improve the patient experience, tackle effectiveness and update practice in the light of evidence from research

Discussion and critical thinking questions

8.1 Think about an organisation with which you are familiar and identify the alignment (or not) of the organisation's values or mission and the culture of the organisation.

8.2 Do you think it is important for an employee's values and the organisational mission to align?

8.3 What part does evidence play in supporting clinical change?

8.4 What part do the NMBA's (2006) *National Competency Standards for the Registered Nurse* play in framing a clinical leader's ability to promote and support change and innovation in practice?

8.5 What part does the clinical leader's own sense of empowerment play in facilitating their participation in proposing or supporting new clinical initiatives?

Learning extension

Think of the clinical environments in which you have worked. Have these envi-ronments always been perfect? Have you ever thought, 'Why are we doing this or that, this way?' Or, 'Why has someone not seen that time, money or energy could be saved by doing things differently?' What has stopped you comment-ing on or suggesting a new or novel approach to doing something differently? If you had the chance to go back to one of these clinical areas, what ideas might you have for doing things differently? How is this approach linked to the actions of a clinical leader?

Further reading

Stanley D. (2011). *Clinical leadership: Innovation into action*. Melbourne: Palgrave Macmillan. This Australian text details an understanding of clinical leadership and the key attributes and skills applied to developing clinical leadership in practice.

References

Acree, C.M. (2006). The relationship between nursing leadership practices and hospital. *Newborn and Infant Nursing Reviews*, 6(1): 34–40.

Anderson, M.A. & Helms, L.B. (2000). Talking about patients: Communication and continuity of care. *Journal of Cardiovascular Nursing*, 14(3): 15–28.

Australian Commission on Safety and Quality in Health Care (ACSQHC) (2011). *Implementation toolkit for clinical handover improvement*. Sydney: ACSQHC.

Avolio, B.J. & Bass, B.M. (1999). Re-examining the components of transformational and transactional leadership using the Multifactor Leadership Questionnaire. *Journal of Occupational & Organizational Psychology*, 72(4): 441–62.

Bennis, W. & Nanus, B. (1985). *Leaders: The strategies for taking charge*. New York: Harper and Row.

Berwick, D. (1994). Eleven worthy aims for clinical leadership of healthcare reform. *JAMA*, 272(10): 797–802.

Bokhour, B.G. (2006). Communication in interdisciplinary team meetings: What are we talking about? *Journal of Interprofessional Care*, 20(4): 349–63.

Burns, J.M. (1978). *Leadership*. New York: Harper and Row.

Clark, L. (2008). Clinical leadership values, beliefs and vision. *Nursing Management*, 15(7): 30–5.

Cook, A. & Holt, L. (2000). *Clinical leadership and supervision*. In D. Dolan & L. Holt (eds), *Accident and emergency theory into practice*. London: Baillière Tindall, pp. 497–503.

Cook, M. (2001a). Clinical leadership that works. *Nursing Management*, 7(10): 24–8.

——(2001b). The attributes of effective clinical nurse leaders. *Nursing Standard*, 15(35): 33–6.

Dean-Barr, S. (1998). Translating clinical leadership into organizational leadership. *Rehabilitation Nursing*, 23(3): 118.

Dignam, D., Duffield, C., Stasa, H., Gray, J., Jackson, D. & Daly, J. (2012). Management and leadership in nursing: An Australian educational perspective. *Journal of Nursing Management*, 20(1): 65–71.

Downey, M., Parslow, S. & Smart, M. (2011). The hidden treasure in nursing leadership: Informal leaders. *Journal of Nursing Management*, 19: 517–21.

Ellis, J.R. & Hartley, C.L. (2009). *Managing and coordinating nursing care*, 5th edn. Philadelphia: Lippincott, Williams & Wilkins.

Goleman, D. (1998). *Working with emotional intelligence*. New York: Bantam Books.

Grohar-Murray, M.E. & Langan, J. (2011). *Leadership and management in nursing*, 4th edn. Boston: Pearson.

Harper, J. (1995). Clinical leadership: Bridging theory and practice. *Nurse Educator*, 20(3): 11–12.

Hein, E.C. (1998). 'Sizing' up the system. In E.C. Hein (ed.), *Contemporary leadership behavior*, 5th edn. Philadelphia: Lippincott, Williams & Wilkins, pp. 295–306.

Huber, D. (2010). *Leadership and nursing care management*, 4th edn. Waltham, MA: Elsevier.

Hurley, J. & Hutchinson, M. (2013). Setting a course: A critical review of the literature on nurse leadership in Australia. *Contemporary Nurse*, 43(2): 178–82.

Jones, L. & Bennett, C.L. (2012). *Leadership in health and social care: An introduction for emerging leaders*. Banbury (UK): Lantern Publishing.

Kean, S., Haycock-Stuart, E., Baggaley, S. & Carson, M. (2011). Followers and the co-construction of leadership. *Journal of Nursing Management*, 19: 507–16.

Kotter, J.P. (1990). *What leaders really do*. Cambridge, MA: Harvard Business School Press.

Lett, M. (2002). The concept of clinical leadership. *Contemporary Nurse*, 12(1): 16–21.

Long, A. (2011). Leadership and management. In T. Swanwick & J. McKimm (eds), *ABC of clinical leadership*. Oxford: Blackwell, pp. 8–13.

MacKian, S. & Simons, J. (2013). *Leading managing caring: Understanding leadership and management in health and social care*. Oxford: Routledge.

Mancini, K. (2015a). Healthcare organizations. In P.S. Yoder-Wise (ed.), *Leading and managing in nursing*, 6th edn. St Louis, MS: Mosby, pp. 118–35.

—— (2015b). Understanding and designing organisational structures. In P.S. Yoder-Wise (ed.), *Leading and managing in nursing*, 6th edn. St Louis, MS: Mosby, pp. 136–52.

Mannix, J., Wilkes, L. & Daly, J. (2013). Attributes of clinical leadership in contemporary nursing: An integrative review. *Contemporary Nurse*, 45(1): 10–21.

McCloskey, J.C., Bulechek, G.M., Moorhead, S. & Daly, J. (1996). Nurses' use and delegation of indirect care interventions. *Nursing Economic$*, 14(1): 22–33.

McCormack, B. & Hopkins, E. (1995). The development of clinical leadership through supported reflective practice. *Journal of Clinical Nursing*, 4(3): 161–8.

McQueen, A.C.H. (2004). Emotional intelligence in nursing work. *Journal of Advanced Nursing*, 47(1): 101–8.

Nursing and Midwifery Board of Australia (NMBA) (2006). National competency standards for the registered nurse. Sydney: NMBA.

Ortega, A., Sánchez-Manzanares, M., Gil, F. & Rico, R. (2013). Enhancing team learning in nursing teams through beliefs about interpersonal context. *Journal of Advanced Nursing*, 69(1): 102–11.

Peach, M. (1995). Reflection on clinical leadership behaviours. *Contemporary Nurse*, 4(1): 33–7.

Rocchiccioli, J.T. & Tilbury, M.S. (1998). *Clinical leadership in nursing*. Philadelphia: W.B. Saunders.

Schneider, P. (1999). Five worthy aims for pharmacy's clinical leadership to pursue in improving medication use. *American Journal of Health System Pharmacy*, 56(24): 2549–52.

Stanley, D. (2006a). Role conflict: Leaders and managers. *Nursing Management*, 13(5): 31–7.

——(2006b). Recognising and defining clinical nurse leaders. *British Journal of Nursing*, 15(2): 108–11.

——(2008). Congruent leadership: Values in action. *Journal of Nursing Management*, 16: 519–24.

——(2011). *Clinical leadership: Innovation into action*. Melbourne: Palgrave Macmillan.

——(2014). Clinical leadership characteristics confirmed. *Journal of Research in Nursing*, 19(2): 118–28.

Stanton, E., Lemer, C. & Mountford, J. (2010). *Clinical leadership: Bridging the divide*. London: Quay Books.

Swanwick, T. & McKimm, J. (2011). *ABC of clinical leadership*. Oxford: Wiley-Blackwell.

Thompson, J. (2012). Transformational leadership can improve workforce competencies. *Nursing Management – UK*, 18(10): 21–4.

UK Department of Health (2007). *Our health our future: NHS, Next stage review*. Interim Report. London: Stationery Office.

Warren, R. (2005). What's the difference between managing and leading? *Transforming Churches*. Retrieved 20 January 2015 from <http://transformingchurch.com/resources/2005/08whats_the_dif.php>.

Wyatt, J. (1995). Hospital information management: The need for clinical leadership. *BMJ*, 311(6998): 175–8.

Zaleznik, A. (1977). Managers and leaders: Are they different? In *Harvard Business Review: On Leadership*. Cambridge, MA: Harvard Business School Press, pp. 61–88.

Contributing to evidence-based healthcare cultures through lifelong learning

9

Lisa Beccaria, Clint Moloney and Craig Lockwood

Learning objectives

- Understand relevant frameworks that relate to research implementation.
- Formulate an understanding of facilitators and barriers to research-utilisation practices.
- Identify the dispositions required for evidence-based practice, teamwork and change management.
- Understand team dynamics relating to effective change management.
- Create an understanding of the associated links between evidence-based healthcare, professional practice and lifelong learning.
- Understand the evolution of skills and knowledge regarding evidence utilisation and leadership.

Key terms

- Change management
- Evidence-based healthcare
- Heterophilous
- Homophilous
- Implementation science
- Lifelong learning
- Personal disposition
- Research utilisation

Introduction

This chapter explores communication issues for future healthcare professionals when contributing to **evidence-based healthcare** cultures through **lifelong learning**. Those training to become clinicians need to understand relevant frameworks guiding evidence **implementation science** and **research utilisation** skills development. Students should be aware of known communication aids and barriers to research utilisation. By understanding the **personal dispositions** that can enable effective **change management**, students will better understand team dynamics. This chapter examines the associated links to professional practice and the evolution of communication skills and knowledge as they relate to evidence utilisation and leadership.

evidence-based healthcare: emphasises the use of evidence from well-designed and conducted research in healthcare decision-making

lifelong learning: the ongoing, voluntary and self-motivated pursuit of knowledge for personal or professional reasons

implementation science: all aspects of research relevant to the scientific study of methods to promote the uptake of research findings into routine settings in clinical, community and policy contexts

research utilisation: the movement of innovative research evidence into practice

personal disposition: the predominant or prevailing tendency of one's own inclinations and preferences

change management: an approach to transitioning individuals, teams and organisations to a desired future state

Understanding theoretical frameworks that guide communication processes and skills development

Using frameworks that can support and guide evidence-based decision-making in lifelong learning is essential for students to be reassured that a particular evidence-based initiative is the right one in a given context. Frameworks like evidence-based practice, integrated risk management, change management and clinical reasoning are important tools for gathering the necessary factors to aid such a decision.

Healthcare professionals from a variety of disciplines realise the value of evidence transfer in evidence-based healthcare practices (Gibson, Martin, & Singer, 2004). Evidence-based practice (EBP) means healthcare professionals use patient evaluation and intervention guidelines for particular disorders and diagnostic-related groups. EBP considers the individual's pathophysiologic knowledge of the disorder(s) being treated, their clinical expertise and the patient's preferences for treatment (Pearson et al., 2005).

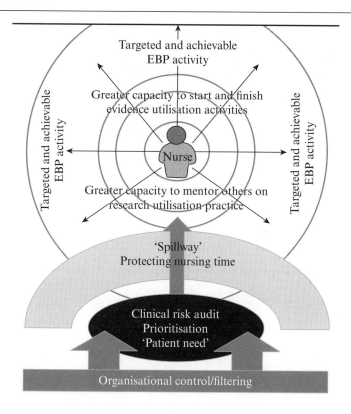

FIGURE
9.1 *Spillway model*

EBP is the careful and sensible use of the best available levels of evidence alongside the clinical expertise of healthcare professionals. To understand the transfer of evidence, students first need to understand the sources of best evidence – for example, published research in healthcare journals. It is also imperative for students to understand the hierarchy of evidence behind best evidence (Averis & Pearson, 2003; Pearson et al., 2005) – for example, the empirical evidence that stems from a randomised control trial or the descriptive perceptual evidence flowing from sound qualitative research. Understanding the source of evidence can also mean a student recognises a gap in the availability of sound evidence (see Figure 9.1). This can also lead to a healthcare decision based solely on expert opinion and years of clinical experience.

TABLE 9.1 *JBI levels of evidence*

LEVEL OF EVIDENCE	FEASIBILITY F (1–4)	APPROPRIATENESS A (1–4)	MEANINGFULNESS M (1–4)	EFFECTIVENESS E (1–4)
1	Metasynthesis of research with unequivocal synthesised findings	Metasynthesis of research with unequivocal synthesised findings	Metasynthesis of research with unequivocal synthesised findings	Meta-analysis (with homogeneity) of experimental studies (e.g. RCT with concealed randomisation) OR One or more large experimental studies with narrow confidence intervals
2	Metasynthesis of research with credible synthesised findings	Metasynthesis of research with credible synthesised findings	Metasynthesis of research with credible synthesised findings	One or more smaller RCTs with wider confidence intervals OR Quasi-experimental studies (without randomisation)
3	(a) Metasynthesis of text/opinion with credible synthesised findings (b) One or more single research studies of high quality	(a) Metasynthesis of text/opinion with credible synthesised findings (b) One or more single research studies of high quality	(a) Metasynthesis of text/opinion with credible synthesised findings (b) One or more single research studies of high quality	(a) Cohort studies (with control group) (b) Case-controlled (c) Observational studies (without control group)
4	Expert opinion	Expert opinion	Expert opinion	Expert opinion, or physiology bench research, or consensus

Source: Joanna Briggs Insitute (2014b)

Healthcare leaders have a duty of care to implement changes that stem from a hierarchy of evidence. Shifting this evidence from knowledge to implementation in clinical practice is dependent on the aptitude of all healthcare professionals to successfully communicate the intentions of implementation, and thereby ensure the long-term sustainability of the changes. However, successful communication is seldom easy to achieve, and changing the mindset of other healthcare professionals poses an ongoing challenge. Healthcare professionals must consider recognised and unrecognised barriers that impact on the transference of this evidence (Moloney, 2013). The digital age has led to additional barriers to accessing information (Moloney & Beccaria, 2009). These barriers are explored in greater depth later in this chapter and were also presented in Chapter 7. The tempo of change within the world of healthcare has also contributed to an overload of new information and a consequent inability to find and retain new information (Brown et al., 2010).

Although implementing new evidence has improved patient care standards in some instances, a gap still exists between the expansion of valued research outcomes and convenient access for healthcare professionals to improve care. Frequently, knowledge and proposed interventions revealed by evidence-based practice research remain largely unshared due to constrained resources and a scarcity of recognised utilisation intent or direction (Averis & Pearson, 2003). Efforts by the Joanna Briggs Institute (JBI) (2014a) have focused on enlarging the extent of work undertaken around increased evidence-based utilisation strategies. Initiatives like JBI Connect Plus have ensured that the needs of health consumers and the activities of research-active health professionals have a common communication platform for evidence-based practice. This modern communication platform is intended to enhance access and improve the effectiveness of strategies when implementing research findings (Metsälä & Vaherkoski, 2014).

Transference models have been well studied in the literature (Estabrooks et al., 2003; Kitson et al., 2008; Pearson et al., 2005; Rogers, 2002). Ironically, very few directly consider personal and organisational communication skills or attributes. However, some – such as the Promoting Action on Research Implementation in Health Services (PARIHS) Model (see Table 9.2) – focus on the interactions between three key elements for implementation, including establishing a context (Kitson et al., 2008). This is important to an individual or team wishing to introduce change, as understanding the willingness of an organisation to embrace change dictates the level and form of communication required to promote effective utilisation. Understanding context is a key attribute to other models, such as the Knowledge-to-Action Framework (Kastner & Straus, 2012; Straus et al., 2008), which advocates for an adaptation of knowledge to the local context. On the other hand, Rogers' (2002) Innovation Diffusion Theory hinges on a scale of likeliness for adoption – that is, from laggards in innovation through to inspired innovators. Integral to these theories is the need to understand social knowledge – for example, the likelihood of effective social interactions with the end-users of evidence.

TABLE 9.2 *Outline of research utilisation models*

SOURCE	DISCUSSION DOMAIN	PROCESS
Crane, 1985; CURN Project, 1981; Closs & Bryar, 2001; Funk et al., 1991	Conduct and Utilisation of Research in Nursing Project (CURN)	› Problem identification › Assess knowledge base › Design practice change/innovation › Conduct clinical trial › Adopt, alter or reject change › Diffuse innovation › Institutional change and maintain innovation over time › Outcome: change in client outcome
Stetler 2001	The Stetler-Marram Model	› Preparation phase › Validation phase › Comparative evaluation phase › Decision-making phase › Translation/application phase › Evaluation phase › Outcome: use of findings in practice
Rogers, 2002	Rogers' Innovation Diffusion Model	Some of the characteristics of each category of adopter include: › innovators – venturesome, educated, multiple info sources, greater propensity to take risk › early adopters – social leaders, popular, educated › early majority – deliberate, many informal social contacts › late majority – sceptical, traditional, lower socio-economic status › laggards – neighbours and friends are main info sources, fear of debt Rogers also proposed a five-stage model for the diffusion of innovation: › Knowledge – learning about the existence and function of the innovation › Persuasion – becoming convinced of the value of the innovation › Decision – committing to the adoption of the innovation › Implementation – putting it to use › Confirmation – the ultimate acceptance (or rejection) of the innovation
Kleiber & Titler, 1998	The Iowa Model of Research in Practice	› Expected outcomes documented › Practice interventions designed › Practice changes implemented › Process and outcomes evaluated › Intervention modified if required › Outcome: improving clinical practice through research

SOURCE	DISCUSSION DOMAIN	PROCESS
Jones, 2000	The Linkage Model	❭ User system ❭ Resource/knowledge-generating system ❭ Transmission mechanism ❭ Feedback mechanism ❭ Outcome: transmission of research ❭ Innovations
Kitson et al., 2008	Promoting Action on Research Implementation in Health Services (PARIHS) Model	This model focuses on the interactions between three key elements for implementation: ❭ Evidence (E) ❭ Context (C) and ❭ Facilitation (F) The model asserts that successful implementation (SI) of evidence into practice has as much to do with the context or setting to which the new evidence is being introduced and how that new evidence is introduced (facilitated into practice) as it has to do with the quality of the evidence.

There are many interpersonal communication process models that can be applied alongside such theories. An individual or group trying to establish a communication channel (the medium by which the message is delivered and received) must therefore understand the context. Barriers to communication can include noise (everything that interferes with an accurate expression or receipt of a message) and feedback (an appropriate reaction from the receiver signifying whether the message has been received in its intended form) (Moloney, 2013; Portoghese et al., 2012). Research focusing on nursing perceptions of research utilisation reveals 'excess noise' in nurses' immediate and surrounding environments that restricts the ability to engage in research utilisation. This constitutes an overload of communication, leaving room for misinterpretation. The Spillway Model (Figure 9.1) highlights the need to better control this excess noise, allowing the end-user of research findings to start and finish research implementations (Moloney, 2013).

Those training to be healthcare professionals (and future leaders) are required to view communication in a different light. A student's knowledge of appropriate communication will be based on a context of experience rather than the application of communication skills and knowledge. For example, the context of a clinical placement in an emergency room may require a different focus of communication to that in a rehabilitation ward. At the core of healthcare professional activity sits irregularity, obscurity and a risk of alternative interpretations

(Rangachari et al., 2014). Thus the topic of evidence-based research utilisation is not stagnant; it has the capacity for transformation through further research – and therefore an individual's or group's lifelong learning. This means the seeds of learning around evidence-based practice and the communication tools required to assist in embedding new evidence need to be planted early for the student's benefit (Lavis, Robertson & Woodside, 2003; Rangachari et al., 2014). In theory, communication flow must occur in two directions. Most transference models make no reference to this two-way communication; rather, they indirectly refer to communication – that is, the Knowledge-to-Action Framework, which considers that users of knowledge need to be included in the action or cyclic decision process to make sure any implementation meets their needs. This implies there is a two-way communication, yet never specifically advocates for it. The PARIHS framework also has an indirect communication loop, indicating that there should be interaction with the stakeholders; however, it does not elaborate on the shape of two-way communication (Kastner & Straus, 2012; Kitson et al., 2008).

Evidence implementation within an organisation requires effective communication strategies. Evidence implementation should presuppose innovation adoption: decisions typically made by senior health managers regarding changes to evidence in practice should include the staff involved in their longitudinal implementation (Rogers, 2002).

Rogers' Diffusion of Innovation theory seems to deliver significant advantages (Table 9.2), enabling an investigation of the true root cause of why a new initiative is either adopted or not adopted, closely mimicking change strategies like the normative-reeducative strategy. The innovation diffusion theory originates from dynamic systems theory, and offers a sound platform when considering the level at which healthcare professionals should engage in research. An appreciation of the important links between theory and practice prepares these future professionals to apply knowledge and skills throughout their careers to facilitate effective change (Rogers, 2002).

Investing energy in the identification and spread of effective evidence-based practice is important. There is a need to make better use of systems like JBI Connect Plus that identify change that is having an impact, and to understand why this has occurred. It is highly recommended that students become familiar with these systems as soon as possible, and make good use of them in assignments. As the leaders of tomorrow, nursing graduates armed with these tools will be well placed to influence the necessary diffusion of new evidence into practice (Metsälä & Vaherkoski, 2014; Pearson et al., 2005). The aim should be to increase the global uptake of evidence-based practice, so receptiveness to change and improvement become built-in features of practice, supported by international, national and organisational-level structures and processes (Pearson et al., 2005).

A 'change agent' is recommended for effective communication in the implementation process. All students training to be part of the wider healthcare workforce should aspire to be such a change agent at one time or another. This person's role is to influence and guide the innovation decision, and they are often external to the organisation. Having an external person driving change can often work in favour of change, as this person can remain neutral throughout the process. Their messages should be targeted to the intended audience for effective adoption of the innovation. A change agent usually has a high degree of expertise in the innovation. They are viewed as effective if they are perceived as credible, competent, reliable and empathetic. A skilled change agent will diagnose problems and determine alternatives to meet adopters' needs, then reinforce and stabilise the new behaviour so they can leave the role of change agent (Rogers, 2002; Woodward et al., 2014). Since they are usually **heterophilous** to the organisation it is important to also have the support of champions and opinion leaders who are **homophilous** (Rogers, 2002; Woodward et al., 2014). Opinion leaders are individuals who have influence on others but not by their formal leadership role. They have large interpersonal communication networks and can be used to positively influence the diffusion of an innovation (Rogers, 2002).

heterophilous: the degree to which pairs of individuals who interact are different with respect to certain attributes, such as beliefs, values, education and social status

homophilous: the degree to which pairs of individuals who interact are similar with respect to certain attributes, such as beliefs, values, education and social status

Research shows healthcare professionals want research engagement to be governed by risk-management prioritisation. They believe there is greater relevance to patient needs and care outcomes when targeting implementation projects (Moloney, 2013). Research also suggests that while it is essential to acknowledge that evidence-based practice adoption needs to be encouraged, recommendations also need to be refined to the patient for whom care is being provided, and the context in which that care is provided (Fallon et al., 2006). Furthermore, it is also important for an innovation to be appropriately refined to the context of the target population (Bowtell et al., 2012). It is clear that individuals or groups who are driving change must keep integrated risk management at the forefront of patient care innovations. Staff members are more likely to embrace change if they can clearly see its worth in relation to improving care standards. If staff members are to recognise and relate to any risk prioritisation, it is essential to communicate risk 'trending' (for example, moderate to high risk) as identified by integrated risk management systems (Vincent, 2006). Risk management and the risk trending that stems from it are valuable tools for the change agent when they need to provide evidence and justification for change.

Understanding known facilitators and barriers to research-utilisation practices

Healthcare professionals have a critical role in fostering optimal patient outcomes, and monitoring and assessing patients is a key element of this. This literature highlights mounting concern around issues of patient safety and risk of harm when a patient's physical condition deteriorates unexpectedly (Henneman, Gawlinski & Giuliano, 2012; Odell, Victor & Oliver, 2009; Preston & Flynn, 2010). Dresser (2012, p. 110) states that 'a turn of events unacknowledged by a healthcare professional can markedly alter the course of a patient's condition and outcome'.

The mismanagement of a patient's healthcare data can result in morbidity and even mortality. However, effective clinical reasoning skills can help a healthcare professional to detect and manage patient deterioration early, thus preventing adverse patient outcomes (Levett-Jones et al., 2010). Healthcare professionals are sometimes reluctant to act on adverse findings or may not know the degree of urgency if they do not understand the physiology involved in the changes they observe in the patient's condition (Levett-Jones et al., 2010; Preston & Flynn, 2010). It is imperative to consider these staff skills in relation to any change. During the implementation of any evidence-based care standards, there will always be a reliance on skilled and knowledgeable healthcare professionals to measure indicators of change. For example, we may wish to understand whether patient recovery time has shortened or patient pain control has been vastly improved. A healthcare professional's clinical reasoning skills therefore play a key role in the communication process throughout any implementation process (Levett-Jones et al., 2010).

Clinical reasoning skills may well present a barrier to change if cyclic patient assessment is not well performed. It is imperative for those driving change to establish the context of known and unknown barriers to change. Communication (or a lack of it) is a well-recognised barrier to change (Levett-Jones et al., 2010; van Bekkum & Hilton, 2013). Physical communication barriers in healthcare can include marked-out territories, 'empires' and circles of trust into which outsiders are not allowed. Closed office doors, barrier screens and divided areas for those of a different status can restrict communication. The larger the work area, the more likely it will be that these barriers may be present. Research shows one of the most significant influences in fostering unified teams is proximity (van Bekkum & Hilton, 2013).

The most likely problem to be encountered when communicating EBP is that everyone sees the world differently and there are various levels of experience. One of the main barriers to unrestricted communication is the emotional barrier. This can be a combination of fear, mistrust and suspicion. The root cause of this emotional block needs to be understood before progressing. Reflecting on one's own emotional intelligence and that of others can unlock potential barriers to change, and thereby improve communication. A facilitator can be used to understand an individual's emotional drivers. Most healthcare professionals are driven by patient-centric care principles because they want what is best for their patient (Davis et al., 2008; van Bekkum & Hilton, 2013).

Behavioural patterns can be 'inherited' due to the close nature of working in a group of healthcare professionals. It is human nature to feel a sense of belonging, and therefore it is easy to become entwined in a culture, regardless of whether it is negative or positive. Defining the context of a given culture can unveil associated cultural barriers and lead to more effective strategies for engagement. There is an increased likelihood of successful implementation within healthcare groups that are happy to accept a change agent, where that change agent is happy to conform to local parameters. However, the likelihood of success becomes lower where there are barriers to a change agent's membership within a collective (Davis et al., 2008; van Bekkum & Hilton, 2013).

Of course, it is difficult to avoid interpersonal barriers and interpersonal conflicts within two-way communication. To decrease the likelihood of conflict, it is best for a change agent to remain flexible and neutral throughout the communication process (Davis et al., 2008; van Bekkum & Hilton, 2013).

The National Institute of Clinical Studies provides a very good overview of mainstream barriers and facilitators that can impact on the EBP implementation process (see Table 9.3). It is highly recommended that a tailored approach designed to analyse likely barriers is considered, as this will aid the change agent in focusing their efforts towards specific barriers (National Institute of Clinical Studies, 2005).

TABLE 9.3 *Types of barriers and enablers that may impede best practice at different levels of healthcare*

LEVEL	TYPE OF BARRIER OR ENABLER	EXAMPLES
The innovation itself	> Advantages in practice > Feasibility > Credibility > Accessibility > Attractiveness	Clinical practice guidelines may be perceived as inconvenient or difficult to use. Guidelines recommending the elimination of an established clinical practice, such as screening for lung cancer with chest x-rays, may be more difficult to follow than guidelines that recommend adding a new behaviour.
Individual professional	> Awareness > Knowledge > Attitude > Motivation to change > Behavioural routines	Clinicians may not agree with a specific guideline or the concept of guidelines in general. Clinicians may not have the motivation to change or may not feel competent to provide specific services, such as counselling about exercise or diet.
Patient	> Knowledge > Skills > Attitude > Compliance	Patients may expect certain services, such as the prescription of antibiotics for upper respiratory tract infections.
Social context	> Opinion of colleagues > Culture of the network > Collaboration > Leadership	Local opinion leaders may encourage the use of forms of care that have not been shown to be effective, such as screening for ovarian or prostate cancer.
Organisational context	> Care processes > Staff > Capacities > Resources > Structures	Burdensome paperwork or poor communication may inhibit provision of effective care.
Economic and political context	> Financial arrangements > Regulations > Policies	Reimbursement systems may promote unnecessary services or discourage best practice.

Source: National Institute of Clinical Studies (2005)

Case study

You are a registered nurse who is new to an organisation. You are currently working in a very busy acute medical/surgical unit. You have noticed that there is great variation in the use of decimal points in drug dosages and the use of measurement descriptors by doctors – for example, mcg or micro. You know from previous experience that these simple differences in prescribing can lead nurses to making a medication error, potentially causing harm to a patient.

Critical reflection

>> Using the theoretical frameworks already provided in this chapter, consider where you could gather evidence to support your desire to bring about positive change.

r organisation is even more so. For example, how well an organisation is re-ourced, whether the new change might 'fit' within current procedures and policies, and how likely it is that a change might be supported and adopted by decision-makers may all be important factors as to whether a new idea can be turned into reality (Schaffer, Sandau & Diedrick, 2013; Tagney & Haines, 2009).

A person's own lack of confidence in appraising and using evidence in prac-tice is another well-established barrier to research utilisation (Wallin, Boström & Gustavsson, 2012). Difficulties may arise in considering how research find-ings could be applied to practice, having a lack of awareness of the range of clini-cal issues in a speciality area, and knowing how care might best be evaluated af-ter practice change (Fink, Thompson & Bonnes, 2005; Gagan & Hewitt-Taylor, 2004). Ritualistic practice means lacking the confidence to change practice (Savage, 2013). It is particularly important for beginning nurses to recognise these knowledge deficits, and to plan towards addressing these gaps over time.

Identifying clinical issues and potential solutions, and communicating these within the healthcare environment, may be challenging. Often the proc-ess involves identifying issues or problems within the clinical setting, and rais-ing questions about the current situation and whether care could be provided more effectively or efficiently (International Council of Nurses, 2012). These clinical issues or questions may be related to an individual health professional's practice, patient healthcare issues or the organisational environment – even a combination of all of these aspects.

It is not uncommon for nurses – particularly when they are transitioning from a student to a nurse – to feel unsure of their practice, knowledge and skills, and they will often rely on observing more experienced nurses. Begin-ning practitioners may then adopt certain practices without always critically thinking about it (Ferguson & Day, 2007). In terms of evidence-based practice, many beginning practitioners also feel limited in influencing change (Ferguson & Day, 2007; Gagan & Hewitt-Taylor, 2004; Gerrish et al., 2008). With more experience, skills and knowledge, the ability to incorporate evidence within clinical practice increases. It is important to learn from experiences by apprais-ing each situation individually, and considering what has been learnt and what could be applicable to future situations.

Nursing knowledge is derived from many sources, yet beginning nurses have been found to place more importance on less formal mechanisms for ac-quiring knowledge (Gerrish et al., 2008; Mills, Field & Cant, 2009). Nursing involves a strong oral culture within which knowledge is often shared from

Case study

You undertake an initial search of the literature and realise that there are some national guidelines on the use of abbreviations, symbols and terminology in prescribing and administering medicines (ACSQHC, 2015). According to this, the doctors' current prescribing habits are not in accordance with evidence best practice. You raise this issue with your nurse unit manager and state that you would like to investigate this issue further with permission, by looking into current risk-management data stemming from incident reports.

Critical reflection

>> How would you approach communication with the nurse unit manager about this issue?

>> Consider some communication tools that would lead to you obtaining the nurse unit manager's support to pursue this issue.

Case study

In your new workplace, you know there have been staff advocating for the use of structured communication when handing over information to others or when a nurse is seeking a patient review from a doctor. You decide to better document the situation and background, undertake an initial assessment and make some recommendations. You do not want to be authoritarian with your communication, but rather engage the nurse unit manager by presenting the facts, allowing them to engage in democratic decision-making once the evidence has been presented. You provide some examples of the discrepancies with prescriptions and the new evidence you have found that should guide practice. You outline that these types of discrepancies have historically led to errors, and that you also suspect some errors may recently have occurred in the clinical area. You say you feel it may be beneficial to determine whether there has been any recent trending stemming from incident reporting and that you feel a chart audit may be of benefit. You then ask the nurse unit manager for some advice and their opinion about the correct course of action to take. They say they are happy for you to look at incident data and to start leading a change of practice.

Critical reflection

>> Who will you need to liaise with on this issue if you are to start an effective process of change management?

Most healthcare organisations have risk managers and even medication safety officers. First, you would need to seek out these individuals and present them with the evidence. The organisation would also have an integrated risk man-agement committee, or perhaps a safe medications group. Presenting the issue with one or both of these committees would be of value. At some stage, you will require some 'buy-in' from the medical officers. This would need to occur beyond just your clinical area, as this issue will no doubt turn out to be broader than just your clinical unit. A meeting with a medical officer who is represented on one of the relevant internal committees and who has an interest in medication safety would be of value. The key to enabling this change in practice in accordance with evidence-based recommendations will be to enable joint support and engage many key stakeholders who would also have an interest in improving medication prescribing.

Understanding the dispositions to enable effective change management

A key emphasis of nursing care is to be patient focused and accountable in providing effective and efficient care. Care should be planned and implemented upon a strong evidence base, while taking into account the practitioner's own clinical expertise and patients' preferences and values. As already highlighted, a wide variety of factors can determine how evidence is translated and utilised at the point of care. While organisational factors play an important role in research utilisation and implementation, individual nurses play an even more critical role. Each nurse has their own inherited or acquired personal dispositions, some of which may contribute towards them becoming an evidence-based practice nurse. These dispositions may encompass attitudinal, behavioural and critical-thinking domains. Individual dispositions can relate to both the adoption of evidence into practice, and act as facilitators of change. Furthermore, some nurses will not only adopt and utilise evidence in practice, but will also actively engage in ways to manage and lead change processes related to practice and organisational change.

Having a positive attitude towards improving patient care and 'making a difference' is considered one of the key pillars of critical practice (Brechin, 2000). Nurses are often best placed to understand patient populations. As a result, they are able to identify issues and develop solutions. Having a shared common goal of wanting to improve care should be fundamental. It has been clearly identified in the literature that a negative attitude towards evidence-based practice is a major barrier when it comes to research utilisation (Fink, Thompson & Bonnes, 2005; Rycroft-Malone et al., 2004), so it is important to have a positive attitude and a belief that evidence-based practice will improve

patient experiences and outcomes (Waters et al., 2009). Esse need to be able to see a clear link between research and implicatic in order to actively engage in evidence-based practice (Rycroft-2004).

Becoming an evidence-based nurse also requires critical thi there are many definitions and descriptions of critical thinking in often these include personal dispositions such as being open-m dent, flexible, inquisitive, information-seeking, reflective, logical cal (Profetto-McGrath et al., 2009; Shoulders, Follett & Eason, 20 steen et al., 2010).

Critical thinking involves gathering and seeking information; and investigating clinical practice; analysing and evaluating vai es of information and knowledge within a clinical context; and b problem-solve and apply theory to practice. This information-gat be from one's own practice or from observing others; there can be i natives to solving an issue, so seeking ideas from others may help. helps to seek out and learn from others who are more experienced. the role of observer is to be expected at the transition phase betwe nursing student and practitioner; however, in order to become an ent critical thinker, it is important to move beyond this curiosity s important to develop heightened critical analysis skills by analysing with existing knowledge, being open-minded to others' ideas and knowledge to fill gaps (Hunter et al., 2014; Shoulders, Follett & Easoi

Being open-minded involves receiving and considering new ideas. ity to actively listen to others and respect their ideas is important. 1 involve other nurses, but may also extend to other roles within a multi nary team environment. It may be that others have previously identifi lar problems and solutions. Sharing ideas can foster a greater sense of within healthcare teams, and often has the advantage of attracting intei support from others, which may transpose to other teamwork situations Bergman & Richards, 2013). Having people feel involved and empow provide their ideas is a key aspect of change management. This can be ac both formally and informally. In formal situations, it might involve rais sues at team meetings and allowing everyone to contribute in a safe and su ive environment. Informally, a discussion in the lunchroom might prove for gauging the thoughts and ideas of others.

While identifying problems or issues is important, developing ide: solutions that fit or are likely to be successfully adopted within a work

those more experienced to those less experienced. This may mean the importance placed upon less formal ways of gaining knowledge, such as through experiential learning and interactions with other health professionals, may be judged more highly than knowledge gained from formal research journals. It is important for those mentoring beginning practitioners to be cognisant of the developmental nature of skills and knowledge, ensuring that the 'knowledge of caring' also incorporates a strong evidence base, or at least identifying where there may be gaps in knowledge (Anderson & Willson, 2009; Beskine, 2009).

Having an overall investigative or curious approach is fundamental in critical thinking and continued lifelong learning (Kedge & Appleby, 2009). Curiosity can stem from an innate thirst or drive for knowledge, or alternatively from the need to address an unpleasant stimulus – for example, experiencing the pressure of not knowing something and potentially feeling embarrassed among colleagues (Kedge & Appleby, 2009).

Reflective thinking is part of critical thinking. This may involve self-reflection of practice, with the goal of developing into a more critical and independent student learner (Ireland, 2008), which should have positive benefits for patient care (Dolphin, 2013). While there are many reflective models to guide nursing practice, their processes are often similar. Many processes begin by identifying and describing something that has happened or is happening, reflecting on the aspects of the situation, analysing the situation (considering other previous situations) and considering new perspectives from learning and considerations for future practice (Mantzoukas, 2008). Sharing these understandings with fellow students and healthcare colleagues has the potential to generate opportunities for further discussion and insights.

Innovation often stems from reflecting on and challenging previous knowledge and practices, including beliefs and attitudes about why things are done the way they are (Matthew-Maich et al., 2010). Within the clinical setting, engaging in reflective thinking can occur as part of a debriefing process, in discussion within professional development workshops or during formalised mentoring relationships (Beskine, 2009; Matthew-Maich et al., 2010).

Another key disposition of becoming an evidence-based nurse is being patient-focused – for example, it is important to be aware of the acquired knowledge the patient brings to a healthcare encounter and to ensure accurate information is provided. While it can be positive for patients to access health information themselves, sometimes this information may not be accurate, and subsequently patients may have high expectations about care. With the ease of access to internet-based healthcare information, patients may already feel they have an understanding of signs, symptoms and treatment options (Rodin et al., 2009). It can be a balancing act to meet the needs of the patient while communicating evidence confidently in a way that respects and maintains the integrity of the relationship (van Bekkum & Hilton, 2013). Where the evidence available is unclear, not of high quality or not contextualised to the patient's situation, the nurse must use skills in not only the critical appraisal of evidence, but in making decisions regarding how and what to present to the patient (van Bekkum & Hilton, 2013). It is an important skill to provide clear rationales to patients. This has to be done by providing information the patient understands but that also considers the patient's context.

Finally, being open to and engaging in change is another key disposition of becoming an evidence-based nurse. While many organisational factors are associated with change, the micro aspects of attitudes – readiness to change, openness to change, commitment to change and cynicism about change – have all been found to be important psychological factors in the change process (Choi, 2011). How change is perceived and responded to may certainly be different for each person. Change attitudes, behaviours and actions may also be dependent upon how the organisation itself supports innovation and change.

The dispositions discussed to date may not just apply to adopting evidence into practice; they may also apply to taking more proactive steps to identify ways to improve patient care and to lead the way for positive change. There is emerging literature on the role of facilitators, change agents and role models in promoting research utilisation (McCormack et al., 2013; Melnyk, 2014). This means leadership, change management and even skills in persuading and empowering others to change are all seen as necessary dispositions for effective research utilisation within the nursing profession.

Understanding team dynamics and effective change management

Studies have further suggested that group membership and dynamics are key factors in developing an evidence-based culture. The global shortage of qualified registered nurses has also been associated with poor quality communication between nurses, leading to reduced team-based problem-solving, a loss of group culture and worse patient outcomes. This is a further indication of the importance of staffing as an opportunity to increase the quality of care (Brunetto et al., 2013). The need for effective evidence-based care practices to be a group activity rather than an individual one is particularly suited to the nursing profession, where team-based care has a long-established history (Brunetto et al., 2013).

The evidence in favour of positive supervisor–nurse relationships, teamwork and well-being is of benefit to employers. It is also of benefit to nurse leaders seeking to develop and enhance the skills and knowledge of staff in their units by providing a stable workplace, as these cultural characteristics explain almost half of nurses' commitment to their hospital or their intentions to leave. These findings suggest a leadership focus on improving the quality of workplace relationships as a first step in retaining skilled nurses. It is also the first crucial step in bringing a culture of evidence to practice settings (Brunetto et al., 2013).

Group membership and workplace culture bring clinical benefits to the ability to evaluate current practice and implement changes to improve or develop a best-practice culture, as the above findings indicate. Evidence supports groups being enabled and empowered to take a problem or issue in practice and work through to a solution where the members of the group have equally valued input and voice (Trowbridge, 2011). While these characteristics are the hallmark of healthy work environments, there is another key layer that characterises good implementation studies, and an evidence-based clinical culture.

Leadership

Leadership has been described as the glue that holds a healthy work environment together (Shirey, 2006). Leadership demonstrated through collaborative practice-led change processes has been shown to have a positive impact on the development of an evidence-based culture. Programs such as the JBI Clinical Fellowship create opportunities for group engagement processes in the work environment, where the outcomes are improved practices and better patient outcomes. To effectively change practice, teams setting up clinical audit projects are using the six identified markers of leadership: skilled communication, true collaboration, effective decision-making, appropriate staffing, meaningful recognition and authentic leadership (Forsythe et al., 2013; Shirey, 2006).

While team dynamics are intrinsic to the whole project, in this case study it is Phase 2 that best demonstrates the capacity of evidence-based quality improvement projects to illustrate how complex concepts such as group productivity, social perceptions, group membership, culture and leadership can best be utilised to achieve improved patient outcomes (Trowbridge, 2011). However,

TABLE 9.4 *Results of the team-based GRiP analysis from JBI-PACES*

BARRIERS	STRATEGIES	RESOURCES
No falls screening tool.	Develop a falls screening tool.	Project lead to develop a tool.
Motivation of nurses to engage in falls screening program.	Ensure regular communication to nurses to promote nurse engagement.	Project lead and CSC to regularly text, email and talk with nurses.
Ensure falls screening tools collected at all sites.	Postbox for screening tools available at all sites.	Project lead developed a postbox, CSC emptied routinely and forwarded tool to project lead.

Source: Trowbridge (2011)

changing practice is complex, requiring the support of a majority of the team, consideration of institutional policy, the types of resources needed to facilitate the change and strategies to make the change sustainable.

In a project on fall prevention and screening, Trowbridge (2011) found that barriers to best practice were identified by group process, where the results of the audit were discussed by staff involved in day-to-day care with management and policy-makers. A team-based approach was essential to this project, with equal consideration given to all ideas and suggestions for practice improvement, leading to consensus on which ideas to target first, and the development of an action plan that would engage each member of the project team.

The structure of JBI-PACES facilitates a situational analysis based on barrier identification, strategy planning, and resource implications for each agreed practice improvement strategy. Following a group process, this project identified a series of barriers and developed strategies for each, together with the resources required to achieve the practice change. As can be seen from Table 9.4, barriers can include not only tools and guides, but subjective issues such as cultural resistance, change fatigue and uptake of new practice requirements.

Cultural influence in communication and nursing practice

Good communication is the basis of effective practice and, as highlighted in this chapter, is also the basis of a healthy work environment. In the clinical audit project that provided the case study data for this section, multi-tiered communication strategies promoted and maintained changes that improved nursing

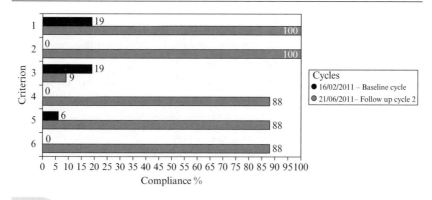

FIGURE
9.2 *Pre- and post-implementation data on percentage of compliance with best practice*

practice and patient care outcomes. The nurses in this project used group meetings to discuss results from the first audit and to develop ideas for how to change practice in positive ways. They also used team-based discussions to develop content for how to present information on practice change to the entire unit, to develop flyers and information, and to address barriers to compliance (Trowbridge, 2011).

As can be seen from Table 9.4, these were strategies that required a whole-of-team level of engagement for the development of a falls screening tool; promotion of the tool to all nurses; regular reminders regarding continued use of the tool; and reminders and processes for storage of completed assessments. The benefits of having a team-based approach to culture change are evident from Figure 9.2, which shows both the baseline and end-of-project outcomes achieved. As illustrated, compliance with best practice was substantially improved. Important to the success of this project was a feedback process that all staff could access throughout the project in order to offer their own thoughts and perspectives on using the assessment tool. Future nurse leaders should regularly ask themselves about the last time they used a feedback process to engage team members in practice-change projects (Trowbridge, 2011).

Figure 9.2 illustrates the impact obtainable in a group-driven process for quality improvement based on evidence. It is important to note that these outcomes were driven by a group-based process founded in open communication and relying upon a team contribution, with equal voice given to all ideas and a consensus-based approach to activities. It could be argued these are normative values in nursing practice, as it is often modelled on team-based approaches.

However, this example also illustrates that team-based nursing can be extended in its scope to implement best practice facilitated in the presence of a positive team dynamic, or group culture, that is enhanced by cultural influences, leadership and effective communication.

If this case study presents evidence and strategies for success in culture shaping, it is important to identify common pitfalls in order to avoid them. Evidence from a series of interviews with nurse leaders found that cultural practices can change when seeking to develop a culture of positive communication that drives and guides practice, but the reasons for change need to be clearly understood and widely accepted. Approaches can and should be specific to the local context, as diversity is reflective of variations in environments, policy constraints and current ward/unit cultures. While the benefits of positive culture change have been linked to healthy work environments, no current data suggest that this needs to be a costly process compared with the benefits gained. Implementing and sustaining cultural change can also be challenging, and strategies need to be tailored to the local environment. Team-based approaches that bring in key stakeholders are a key way to strengthen any project. Education and staff development are also critical, yet these strategies have resource implications, as they may take nurses away from bedside care; therefore, leadership support is essential (Shield et al., 2013).

Links to professional practice

As outlined in previous chapters, nurses in Australia abide by various codes, standards and competencies, laws, policies and procedures, and nursing frameworks and theories. Undergraduate nursing curricula have the underlying goal of providing opportunities to develop future healthcare professionals who have the knowledge, skills, behaviours, attitudes and ways of thinking that will best prepare them for a complex, diverse and ever-changing healthcare environment. In this sense, students are being prepared to engage in professional practice, so it is necessary to define exactly what this is.

Before we look at professional practice, let's consider what is meant by the term 'professional'. Typically, a professional is someone whose job requires them to have special education, training, skills and qualifications to be able to perform their work competently and safely. In addition, the person may have been judged by others as being competent against a set of standards.

If we then examine the characteristics of a profession, we can see that this becomes broader. Hammer (2000) describes a professional or a profession as having both structural and attitudinal attributes. Examples of structural attributes may include aspects such as having a specialised body of theory, knowledge and skills, codes of ethics and autonomy. Attitudinal attributes refer to aspects such as a belief in service to others, having a sense of calling to that profession and helping others, and the ability to make professional decisions regardless of external pressures from others (Hammer, 2000). It is also suggested that professionals will put their patients' needs above their own as an altruistic disposition (Hammer, 2000; Wood, 2014).

Wood (2014) suggests that nurses need to have the intelligence to be able to learn, analyse and process information, but also the desire to help others and an intrinsic passion for caring. When it comes to nursing leadership, this extends to technical and practical skills to provide competent care, building capacity within teams, being supportive of others, having effective communication skills, having a team focus, being a role model and having evidence-based rationales (Mannix, Wilkes & Daly, 2013).

A definition of nursing provided by the International Council of Nurses gives a comprehensive view of the diversity of roles, responsibilities and patients in different developmental stages, circumstances and settings from across the health/illness continuum:

> Nursing encompasses autonomous and collaborative care of individuals of all ages, families, groups and communities, sick or well and in all settings. Nursing includes the promotion of health, prevention of illness, and the care of ill, disabled and dying people. Advocacy, promotion of a safe environment, research, participation in shaping health policy and in patient and health systems management, and education are also key nursing roles. (International Council of Nurses, 2014)

This definition highlights the multidimensional nature of the profession of nursing. It also emphasises nurses' autonomy in making decisions. However, Ellis and Standing (2011, p. 6) state that it is 'no longer good enough for nurses to claim they know best for their patients just because they are nurses'. This means nurses increasingly need to justify what they do and how they do it, and be accountable for their activities and patient outcomes (Ellis & Standing, 2011). Part of autonomy is being accountable for one's actions, and this is considered an attribute of being a 'good nurse' (Begley, 2010). While numerous perspectives exist on what accountability means within the context of nursing, a more recent definition encompasses key aspects. Nursing accountability is defined by Krautscheid (2014, p. 46) as:

> taking responsibility for one's nursing judgments, actions, and omissions as they relate to lifelong learning, maintaining competency, and upholding both

quality patient care outcomes and standards of the profession while being answerable to those who are influenced by one's nursing practice.

Intrinsic to the development and actioning of judgements is the ability to think critically. As previously discussed, being a critical thinker is a key disposition of being an evidence-based nurse and a competent nurse under the Australian Nursing and Midwifery Council's *National Competency Standards for the Registered Nurse*. Within these competency standards, the domain of critical thinking and analysis relates in part to the value of evidence and research for practice. As critical thinking in its simplest terms may be considered as 'thinking about one's own thinking', nurses need to reflect on the purpose of their thinking. They also need to consider their level of knowledge; their biases, assumptions, values and beliefs; the information needed to address any gaps in knowledge; and the identification and evaluation of alternatives (Levett-Jones & Bellchambers, 2011).

When it comes to evidence-based practice, critical thinking may take several forms. Levett-Jones and Bellchambers (2011) outline various aspects of critical thinking, including using divergent thinking (the ability to weigh up the importance of information), reasoning (the ability to discriminate between facts and guesses), clarification (noting similarities and differences in information) and reflection (a purposeful activity designed to critically examine how and why things are done and how one's actions impact on others). All of these processes are critical for the nursing process in terms of planning, implementing and evaluating care.

Many stages of an evidence-based approach mirror the nursing process. The first stage of the nursing process is assessment (Ellis & Standing, 2011; Levett-Jones & Bellchambers, 2011). In evidence-based practice, the first step is to identify a problem. This may involve gathering information, making observations and deciphering relevant and irrelevant data. This process often relies heavily on the nurse's communication skills in gathering data, building a rapport and asking open questions to identify key issues. Building relationships is critical to both processes. This may involve the patients themselves, but can also extend to family, friends and other health professionals who have direct care responsibilities.

At times, we seek ways to use evidence to avoid or prevent harm in client populations – for example, using screening tools to assess the risk of in-patient falls (Graham, 2012), or to improve patient care in areas such as asthma management (Chiang et al., 2012; Swerczek et al., 2013). The nurse should consider the best evidence for both the condition and circumstances of the patient, particularly when it comes to planning care. We often seek to gain evidence that helps guide our clinical decision-making by providing a rationale for what we are doing.

While individual nurses can seek out this information, the benefit of sharing this knowledge with colleagues cannot be understated. Learning about how best to plan and implement care on the basis of one patient has the potential to transfer to specific patient populations in a clinical area, thus having the potential to benefit others. Within the clinical area, there may be other staff who would be interested in improving care. Engaging staff in evidence-based practices is more likely when they can listen to and understand the risks to patient safety if practice is not changed.

The evolution of skills and knowledge as they relate to evidence utilisation and leadership

Evidence-based healthcare has been the dominant paradigm within health since the early 1990s. From emerging methods of systematic review to increasingly sophisticated tools and resources in nursing, medicine and allied health, the methods for evidence-based healthcare have been defined, refined and adapted to fit the continuum of care from primary care to acute tertiary sector interventions, as well as residential aged-care sectors and palliative care (Joanna Briggs Institute, 2014a). While some proponents continue to talk about and advocate for evidence-based nursing, evidence-based medicine or other discipline-specific fields of practice, there is a far stronger rationale for all health professionals to take a patient-centred care approach, and therefore focus on evidence-based healthcare as a process that is inclusive of all professions who care for patients (Joanna Briggs Institute, 2014a). After all, patients are much more interested in their healthcare outcomes than which profession has the largest library of evidence. In spite of the perceived distinction between professions related to evidence, there are also remarkable similarities in how the evidence-based clinician is perceived (Harrison et al., 2013; Lou & Durando, 2008).

A clear set of defined activities has emerged as integral to the development of evidence-based healthcare professionals equipped with the knowledge and skills to provide high-quality, up-to-date, evidence-informed clinical practice (Joanna Briggs Institute, 2014a). Students aspiring to be healthcare professionals should therefore demonstrate an ability to:

- develop answerable questions from issues or problems that arise in day-to-day care and decision-making

- search for and identify evidence relevant to the patient from databases and other sources
- critically read and evaluate published evidence for internal and external validity
- implement the evidence in a way that is both effective and appropriate to the contextual needs of the patient
- evaluate the impact of evidence on patient and healthcare outcomes.

These generic 'steps' have been extensively written about over the past two decades. However, opinions diverge regarding the need to understand research (in order to evaluate its quality and relevance), with some advocating for clinicians to be research-savvy practitioners who 'do' research. This needs to be considered in curriculum design for any students aspiring to be part of the global healthcare profession. Patricia Benner's seminal work on novice to expert pathways highlights the value of expert nurses remaining at the bedside, providing care; yet nursing as a profession has continued to dilute and disregard the value of clinicians providing clinical care (Benner, Kyriakidis & Stannard, 2011). Evidence-based healthcare is not an argument for more nurse researchers; it is a way of assisting nurses to better integrate and use evidence in decision-making, and to provide clinical care. Nurse training should therefore encourage and target consistent application of evidence as part of student nurses' clinical and theoretical experience.

One example of this is the focus on skills to better inform decision-making: this is the central basis of evidence-based healthcare, but it has often been confused with a need to *participate* in research, rather than recognising and developing nursing students who are experts in using evidence. Therefore, undergraduate nursing curricula should include a focus on reflection in terms of becoming research *consumers* rather than research *producers*. Reflection on action is an effective strategy for building evidence into our decision-making.

Students tend to absorb some of the culture and work practices of clinical placement settings. Thinking back on the models for evidence-based healthcare described earlier in the chapter, it is useful as students to consider what sources of information are used during the undergraduate program, and reflect on what they feel confident in applying in terms of evidence for best practice. While it can be useful and appropriate to draw on the knowledge and experience of expert clinicians (an important source of discipline knowledge), the knowledge gained can be highly context-specific. It is not uncommon for students to experience advice or instruction that is quite different across clinical placements, even though the activity is the same. How do we balance these kinds of variations in the context of learning and applying best practice?

This chapter is not a call for less nursing research, nor does it advocate that nurses stop being involved in research or building their own professional knowledge base. Rather, these are deemed to be essential activities that ensure patient care is informed by the best available evidence. Coupled with this is a need for students to learn how to access quality evidence. As an example, student nurses need to learn how to appraise sources of information based on relevance and appropriateness, rather than choosing evidence that is most convenient. The following list ranks sources of information from lowest to highest based on convenience:

Convenience

- an expert clinician in a unit/ward at the same point in time
- Wikipedia or Google/Google Scholar
- the Joanna Briggs Institute
- the Cochrane Library.

However, if we rank these resources based on reliability of evidence, resources such as Wikipedia and even expert nurse opinion will be carefully considered when measured against the evidence already available; therefore a ranking would look more like:

Reliability

- the Joanna Briggs Institute
- the Cochrane Library
- other evidence sources (Wikipedia and Google Scholar do not meet the criteria for an evidence-based resource).

The expert nurse has been left off the list – not by accident, but to indicate that they have a different role. Evidence has to be contextualised for local practice environments. This is arguably where the expert nurse fits in: as a senior user of evidence. This should be one of the few reasonable explanations for why the same practice can and does vary between different clinical placements. Being able to recognise good sources of evidence, and to bring that evidence in to our thinking and planning for care, are lifelong skills that will add value to the individual progressing through their undergraduate program, and the profession of nursing as a whole.

If we accept that evidence-based healthcare requires informed decision-making, reflection on action and (in the case of evidence-based practice) reflection on our sources of evidence or information for practice, how we apply them to clinical care (with the advice and leadership of local expert nurses) does demonstrate a high level of evidence awareness. Nursing students with these attributes will be the future leaders of the nursing profession.

The concepts in this chapter cut across the translational healthcare cycle, and can readily be illustrated through a case study-based approach. The following case study excerpts demonstrate the development of an evidence-based culture through a practice change project that is grounded in a collaborative, positive culture-driven workplace. Phase 1 of the project was the establishment phase. As will be shown, evidence supports the importance of a preparatory stage that deals with known barriers and facilitators to the collaborative method before the commencement of the formal project plan (Trowbridge, 2011).

Case study

An evidence-based clinical audit project was undertaken to develop sustainable processes for intervention and prevention advice and support to adults in the community who had been assessed as being at risk of falls. The first phase of the project commenced with a baseline clinical audit to determine current levels of compliance with best practice. The second phase was the most intensive, complex phase. In Phase 2, clinical fellows brought together teams within their workplace to work through a guided process in evaluating issues with current practice, including policy, practice, workplace culture and environment, teamwork, communication and leadership in order to create a consensus evidence-based quality improvement program that engaged all stakeholders. The third phase involved a repeat audit to measure the impact of all change strategies.

In this project, conducted through the Royal District Nursing Service in South Australia, the baseline audit measured current practice against six criteria across 16 patients. The criteria were:

>> All falls and fall interventions are clearly documented in the client's health record.

>> Falls assessment is completed using a falls assessment tool.

>> Falls interventions are tailored to the individual based on their risk assessment.

>> Older community-dwelling adults have received education on reducing risk factors for falls.

>> Community-dwelling adults with a history of falls have received information on home safety interventions.

>> Older community-dwelling adults have received education regarding exercise programs.

Preparing and undertaking clinical audits of complex care needs constitute a team-based process, involving: encouraging buy-in to the project; identifying and establishing the team members; communicating the purpose and methods of the project; obtaining organisational permission; and team leadership. The ability of the nurse leading the set-up process to understand and lead on these aspects of team dynamics is an indicator of how successful the crucial first phase of the project will be. There is good evidence to support and inform the way communication has a positive impact on nursing practice. Equally, there is evidence indicating the risks to patient care and outcomes when communication is poor. The notion of a healthy work environment is now an evidence-based quality indicator that is demonstrated by the presence of skilled communication, equality in collaboration, effectiveness in decision-making, adequacy in staffing and effective clinical leadership (Vaughan & Slinger, 2013). Vaughan and Slinger (2013) found that communication, collaboration and leadership in the presence of appropriate staffing models constituted a healthy work environment, due to the significant benefit to workplace culture.

Summary

Research utilisation and transference models guide the transfer of knowledge between evidence into practice, and provide insight into the communication skills and strategies required. These are necessary to engage in critical dialogue with colleagues, which involves logical reasoning with a clear patient focus. As these processes involve change, it is important to be aware of the barriers to and enablers for change, as well as your own dispositions and strengths. To progress potential improvements in patient care, and because research utilisation is seldom an individual activity, it is important to identify others with whom you can openly discuss and share ideas, and who can be influential as change agents.

Discussion and critical thinking questions

9.1 There are many barriers to nurses implementing evidence-based practice. What are some of these, and how could an individual nurse address them to best facilitate EBP?

9.2. How can student nurses help create a culture of embracing evidence-based practice within a learning environment with other students?

Learning extension

Think of your own personal barriers and enablers for research utilisation, as well as personal dispositions. Develop a table listing these different aspects, and identify key strategies to foster a culture of evidence-based practice to address personal barriers.

Further reading

Open access journal articles

Evidence-Based Behavioral Practice (EBBP) (2015). Bridging research and practice. Retrieved 25 January 2015 from <http://www.ebbp.org>. This is a website designed to help bridge the divide between behavioural health research and practice. It is multidisciplinary, and includes nursing links to evidence-based resources and training resources.

Makic, M.B.F., Martin, S.A., Burns, S., Philbrick, D. & Rauen, C. (2013). Putting evidence into nursing practice: Traditional practices not supported by the evidence. American Association of Critical Care Nurses. Retrieved 25 January 2015 from <http://www.aacn.org/wd/Cetests/media/C1322.pdf>. On this website is a link to an article which provides examples of four nursing practices that, if changed using evidence, could significantly improve patient care.

Squires, J.E., Estabrooks, C.A., Gustavsson, P. & Wallin, L. (2011). Individual determinants of research utilisation by nurses: A systematic review update. Implementation Science. Retrieved 25 January 2015 from <http://www.implementationscience.com/content/6/1/1>.

References

Anderson, J. & Willson, P. (2009). Knowledge management: Organizing nursing care knowledge. *Critical Care Nursing Quarterly*, 32(1): 1–9.

Australian Commission on Safety and Quality in Health Care (ACSQHC) (2015). Medication administration. Retrieved 28 January 2015 from <http://www.safetyandquality.gov.au/our-work/medication-safety/medication-administration>.

Averis, A. & Pearson, A. (2003). Filling the gaps: Identifying nursing research priorities through the analysis of completed systematic reviews. *JBI Reports, International Journal of Evidence-based Healthcare*, 1(3): 49–126.

Begley, A. (2010). On being a good nurse: Reflections on the past and preparing for the future. *International Journal of Nursing Practice*, 16(6): 525–32.

Benner, P., Kyriakidis, P. & Stannard, D. (2011). *Clinical wisdom and intervention in acute and critical care*, 2nd edn. New York: Springer.

Beskine, D. (2009). Mentoring students: Establishing effective working relationships. *Nursing Standard*, 23(30): 35–40.

Bowtell, L., Moloney, C., Kist, A., Parker, V., Maxwell, A. & Reedy, N. (2012). Enhancing nursing education with remote access laboratories. *International Journal of Online Engineering*, 8: 52–9.

Brechin, A. (2000). Introducing critical practice. In A. Brechin, H. Brown & M. Eby (eds), *Critical practice in health and social care*. London: Sage.

Brown, C., Ecoff, L., Kim, S., Wickline, M., Rose, B., Klimpel, K. & Glaser, D. (2010). Multi-institutional study of barriers to research utilisation and evidence-based practice among hospital nurses. *Journal of Clinical Nursing*, 19(13/14): 1944–51.

Brunetto, Y., Shriberg, A., Farr-Wharton, R., Shacklock, K., Newman, S. & Dienger, J. (2013). The importance of supervisor–nurse relationships, teamwork, wellbeing, affective commitment and retention of North American nurses. *Journal of Nursing Management*, 21(6): 827–37.

Chiang, L., Wen, T., Tien, C. & Huang, J. (2012). Evidence-based management of acute asthma exacerbation in children. *Journal of Nursing*, 59(1): 16–23.

Choi, M. (2011). Employees' attitudes toward organizational change: A literature review. *Human Resource Management*, 50(4): 479–500.

Closs, S. & Bryar, R. (2001). The barriers scale: Does it 'fit' the current NHS research culture? *NT Research*, 6: 853–65.

Crane, J. (1985) Research utilisation: Nursing models. *Western Journal of Nursing Research*, 7: 494–7.

CURN Project (1981). *Using research to improve nursing practice*. New York: Grune & Stratton.

Davis, J., Zayat, E., Urton, M., Belgum, A. & Hill, M. (2008). Communicating evidence in clinical documentation. *Australian Occupational Therapy Journal*, 55(4): 249–55.

Dolphin, S. (2013). How nursing students can be empowered by reflective practice. *Mental Health Practice*, 16(9): 20–3.

Dresser, S. (2012). The role of nursing surveillance in keeping patients safe. *Journal of Nursing Administration*, 42(7/8): 361–8.

Ellis, P. & Standing, M. (2011). *Evidence-based practice in nursing*. Exeter: Learning Matters.

Estabrooks, C.A., Floyd, J.A., Scott-Findlay, S., O'Leary, K.A. & Gushta, M. (2003). Individual determinants of research utilization: A systematic review. *Journal of Advanced Nursing*, 43(5): 506–20.

Fallon, T., Buikstra, E., Cameron, M., Hegney, D., Mackenzie, D., March, J. & Pitt, J. (2006). Implementation of oral health recommendations into two residential aged care facilities in a regional Australian city. *International Journal of Evidence-Based Healthcare*, 4(3): 162–79.

Ferguson, L. & Day, A. (2007). Challenges for new nurses in evidence-based practice. *Journal of Nursing Management*, 15(1): 107–13.

Fink, R., Thompson, C. & Bonnes, D. (2005). Overcoming barriers and promoting the use of research in practice. *Journal of Nursing Administration*, 35(3): 121–9.

Forsythe, T., Funari, T., Mayfield, M., Thoms, W., Smith, K., Bradstreet, H. & Scott, P. (2013). Using evidence-based leadership initiatives to create a healthy nursing work environment. *Dimensions of Critical Care Nursing*, 32(4): 166–73.

Funk, S., Champagne, M., Wiese, R. & Tornquist, E. (1991). Barriers to using research findings in practice: The clinician's perspective. *Applied Nursing Research*, 4: 90–5.

Gagan, M. & Hewitt-Taylor, J. (2004). Professional issues: The issues for nurses involved in implementing evidence in practice. *British Journal of Nursing*, 13(20): 1216–20.

Gerrish, K., Ashworth, P., Lacey, A. & Bailey, J. (2008). Developing evidence-based practice: Experiences of senior and junior clinical nurses. *Journal of Advanced Nursing*, 62(1): 62–73.

Gibson, J., Martin, D. & Singer, P. (2004). Setting priorities in healthcare organisations: Criteria, processes, and parameters of success. *BMC Health Services Research*, 4: 25. Retrieved 20 January 2014 from <http://www.biomedcentral.com/1472-6963/4/25>.

Graham, B.C. (2012). Examining evidence-based interventions to prevent inpatient falls. *MEDSURG Nursing*, 21(5): 267–70.

Hammer, D. (2000). Professional attitudes and behaviors: The 'As and Bs' of professionalism. *American Journal of Pharmaceutical Education*, 64: 455–64.

Harrison, M., Graham, I., van den Hoek, J., Dogherty, E., Carley, M. & Angus, V. (2013). Guideline adaptation and implementation planning: A prospective observational study. *Implementation Science*, 8(49): 14. Retrieved 20 January 2015 from <http://www.implementationscience.com/content/8/1/49>.

Henneman, E.A., Gawlinski, A. & Giuliano, K.K. (2012). Surveillance: A strategy for improving patient safety in acute and critical care units. *Critical Care Nurse*, 32(2): e9–e18.

Hunter, S., Pitt, V., Croce, N. & Roche, J. (2014). Critical thinking skills of undergraduate nursing students: Description and demographic predictors. *Nurse Education Today*, 34(5): 809–14.

International Council of Nurses (2012). Closing the gap: From evidence to action. Retrieved 28 January 2015 from <http://www.icn.ch/publications/2012-closing-the-gap-from-evidence-to-action>.

——(2014). Definition of nursing. Retrieved 28 January 2015 from <http://www.icn.ch/who-we-are/icn-definition-of-nursing>.

Ireland, M. (2008). Assisting students to use evidence as a part of reflection on practice. *Nursing Education Perspectives*, 29(2): 90–3.

Irwin, M., Bergman, R. & Richards, R. (2013). The experience of implementing evidence-based practice change: A qualitative analysis. *Clinical Journal of Oncology Nursing*, 17(5): 544–9.

Joanna Briggs Institute (2014a). *2014 Reviewers Manual*. Adelaide: Joanna Briggs Institute. Retrieved 20 January 2015 from <http://joannabriggs.org/assets/docs/sumari/ReviewersManual-2014.pdf>.

—— (2014b). Levels of evidence. Retrieved 28 January 2015 from <http://joannabriggs.org/jbi-approach.html#tabbed-nav=Levels-of-Evidence>.

Jones, J. (2000). Performance improvement through clinical research utilization: The linkage model. *Journal of Nursing Care Quarterly*, 15(1): 49–54.

Kastner, M. & Straus, S. (2012). Application of the knowledge-to-action and medical research council frameworks in the development of an osteoporosis clinical decision support tool. *Journal of Clinical Epidemiology*, 65(11): 1163–70.

Kedge, S. & Appleby, B. (2009). Promoting a culture of curiosity within nursing practice. *British Journal of Nursing*, 18(10): 635–7.

Kitson, A., Rycroft-Malone, J., Harvey, G., McCormack, B., Seers, K. & Titchen, A. (2008). Evaluating the successful implementation of evidence into practice using the PARiHS framework: Theoretical and practical challenges. *Implementation Science*, 3: 1–12.

Kleiber, C. & Titler, M. (1998). Evidence based practice and the revised Iowa Model. Paper presented to Fifth National Research Utilisation Conference, Iowa City, IA, 23–24 April.

Krautscheid, L. (2014). Defining professional nursing accountability: A literature review. *Journal of Professional Nursing*, 30(1): 43–7.

Lavis, J., Robertson, D. & Woodside, J. (2003). How can research organisations more effectively transfer research knowledge to decision makers? *Milbank Quarterly*, 81: 221–48.

Levett-Jones, T. & Bellchambers, H. (2011). *Medical-surgical nursing: Critical thinking in client care*. Sydney: Pearson.

Levett-Jones, T., Hoffman, K., Dempsey, J., Jeong, S., Noble, D. et al. (2010). The 'five rights' of clinical reasoning: An educational model to enhance nursing students' ability to identify and manage clinically 'at risk' patients. *Nurse Education Today*, 30(6): 515–20.

Lou, J. & Durando, P. (2008). *Asking clinical questions and searching for the evidence*. NJ: Thorofare.

Mannix, J., Wilkes, L. & Daly, J. (2013). Attributes of clinical leadership in contemporary nursing: An integrative review. *Contemporary Nurse*, 45(1): 10–21.

Mantzoukas, S. (2008). A review of evidence-based practice, nursing research and reflection: Levelling the hierarchy. *Journal of Clinical Nursing*, 17(2): 214–23.

Matthew-Maich, N., Ploeg, J., Jack, S. & Dobbins, M. (2010). Transformative learning and research utilization in nursing practice: a missing link? *Worldviews on Evidence-Based Nursing*, 7(1): 25–35.

McCormack, B., Rycroft-Malone, J., DeCorby, K., Hutchinson, A.M., Bucknall, T., Kent, B. et al. (2013). A realist review of interventions and strategies to promote evidence-informed healthcare: A focus on change agency. *Implementation Science*, 8(1): 1–12.

Melnyk, B. (2014). Building cultures and environments that facilitate clinician behavior change to evidence-based practice: What works? *Worldviews on Evidence-Based Nursing*, 11(2): 79–80.

Metsälä, E. & Vaherkoski, U. (2014). Medication errors in elderly acute care: A systematic review. *Scandinavian Journal of Caring Sciences*, 28(1): 12–28.

Mills, J., Field, J. & Cant, R. (2009). The place of knowledge and evidence in the context of Australian general practice nursing. *Worldviews on Evidence-Based Nursing*, 6(4): 219–28.

Moloney, C.W. (2013). Behavioural intention and user acceptance of research evidence for Queensland nurses: Provision of solutions from the clinician. *Nurse Education in Practice*, 13(4): 310–16.

Moloney, C. & Beccaria, L. (2009). Perceived facilitators and inhibitors for the use of personal digital assistants (PDAs) by nurses: A systematic review. *JBI Library of Systematice Reviews*, 7(33). Retrieved 20 January 2015 from <http://joannabriggslibrary.org/index.php/jbisrir/article/view/214>.

National Institute of Clinical Studies (2005). Identifying barriers to evidence uptake. Retrieved 28 January 2015 from <http://www.nhmrc.gov.au/_files_nhmrc/publications/attachments/nic55_identifying_barriers_to_evidence_uptake.pdf>.

Odell, M., Victor, C. & Oliver, D. (2009). Nurses' role in detecting deterioration in ward patients: Systematic literature review. *Journal of Advanced Nursing*, 65(10): 1992–2006.

Pearson, A., Wiechula, R., Court, A. & Lockwood, C. (2005). The JBI model of evidence-based healthcare. *International Journal of Evidence-Based Healthcare*, 3(8): 207–15.

Portoghese, I., Galletta, M., Battistelli, A., Saiani, L., Penna, M.P. & Allegrini, E. (2012). Change-related expectations and commitment to change of nurses: The role of leadership and communication. *Journal of Nursing Management*, 20(5): 582–91.

Preston, R. & Flynn, D. (2010). Observations in acute care: Evidence-based approach to patient safety. *British Journal of Nursing*, 19(7): 442–7.

Profetto-McGrath, J., Smith, K.B., Hugo, K., Patel, A. & Dussault, B. (2009). Nurse educators' critical thinking dispositions and research utilization. *Nurse Education in Practice*, 9(3): 199–208.

Rangachari, P., Madaio, M., Rethemeyer, R.K., Wagner, P., Hall, L., Roy, S. & Rissing, P. (2014). Role of communication content and frequency in enabling evidence-based practices. *Quality Management in Healthcare*, 23(1): 43–58.

Rodin, G., Zimmermann, C., Mayer, C., Howell, D., Katz, M. et al. (2009). Clinician–patient communication: Evidence-based recommendations to guide practice in cancer. *Current Oncology*, 16(6): 42–9.

Rogers, E.M. (2002). Diffusion of preventive innovations. *Addictive Behaviors*, 27(6): 989–93.

Rycroft-Malone, J., Harvey, G., Seers, K., Kitson, A., McCormack, B. & Titchen, A. (2004). An exploration of the factors that influence the implementation of evidence into practice. *Journal of Clinical Nursing*, 13(8): 913–24.

Savage, M. (2013). Communicating with haematology patients: A reflective account. *Nursing Standard*, 28(4): 37–43.

Schaffer, M.A., Sandau, K.E. & Diedrick, L. (2013). Evidence-based practice models for organisational change: Overview and practical applications. *Journal of Advanced Nursing*, 69(5): 1197–1209.

Shield, R., Looze, J., Tyler, D., Lepore, M. & Miller, S. (2013). Why and how do nursing homes implement culture change practices? Insights from qualitative interviews in a mixed methods study. *Journal of Applied Gerontology*, 19: 737–63.

Shirey, M. (2006). Authentic leaders creating healthy work environments for nursing practice. *American Journal of Critical Care*, 15(3): 256–67.

Shoulders, B., Follett, C. & Eason, J. (2014). Enhancing critical thinking in clinical practice: Implications for critical and acute care nurses. *Dimensions of Critical Care Nursing*, 33(4): 207–14.

Stetler, C. (2001). Updating the Stetler model of research utilisation to facilitate evidence-based practice. *Nursing Outlook*, 49(6): 272–9.

Straus, S.E., Graham, I.D., Taylor, M. & Lockyer, J. (2008). Development of a mentorship strategy: A knowledge translation case study. *Journal of Continuing Education in the Health Professions*, 28(3): 117–22.

Swerczek, L., Banister, C., Bloomberg, G., Bruns, J., Epstein, J. et al. (2013). A telephone coaching intervention to improve asthma self-management behaviors. *Pediatric Nursing*, 39(3): 125–45.

Tagney, J. & Haines, C. (2009). Using evidence-based practice to address gaps in nursing knowledge. *British Journal of Nursing*, 18(8): 484–9.

Trowbridge, K. (2011). Falls screening and prevention among adults in the community setting with a previous history of falls: A best practice implementation and evidence utilisation project. *JBI Clinical Fellows Monograph*, 2: 282–9.

van Bekkum, J.E. & Hilton, S. (2013). The challenges of communicating research evidence in practice: Perspectives from UK health visitors and practice nurses. *BMC Nursing*, 12(1): 17–25.

Vaughan, L. & Slinger, T. (2013). Building a healthy work environment: A nursing resource team perspective. *Nursing Leadership*, 26(Spec No 70–7): 70–7.

Vincent, C. (2006). *The essentials of patient safety*. Retrieved 24 January 2015 from <http://www.chfg.org/wp-content/uploads/2012/03/Vincent-Essentials-of-Patient-Safety-2012.pdf>.

Wallin, L., Boström, A. & Gustavsson, J. (2012). Capability beliefs regarding evidence-based practice are associated with application of EBP and research use: Validation of a new measure. *Worldviews on Evidence-Based Nursing*, 9(3): 139–48.

Wangensteen, S., Johansson, I.S., Björkström, M.E. & Nordström, G. (2010). Critical thinking dispositions among newly graduated nurses. *Journal of Advanced Nursing*, 66(10): 2170–81.

Waters, D., Crisp, J., Rychetnik, L. & Barratt, A. (2009). The Australian experience of nurses' preparedness for evidence-based practice. *Journal of Nursing Management*, 17(4): 510–18.

Wood, C. (2014). Choosing the 'right' people for nursing: Can we recruit to care? *British Journal of Nursing*, 23(10): 528–30.

Woodward, A., Fyfe, M., Handuleh, J., Patel, P., Godman, B., Leather, A. & Finlayson, A. (2014). Diffusion of e-health innovations in 'post-conflict' settings: A qualitative study on the personal experiences of health workers. *Human Resources for Health*, 12(1): 1–21.

Glossary

academic argument a well-developed, well-structured and well-supported piece of formal writing that persuades the reader to your point of view

accreditation a process by which an assessing entity (for example, a professional body) evaluates the credibility, reliability and validity of a program (such as an educational program) presented by another party for the purposes of approving its fitness for purpose

change management an approach to transitioning individuals, teams and organisations to a desired future state

chronemics non-verbal communication relating to how time is interpreted

clinical leadership putting clinicians at the heart of shaping and running clinical services to deliver excellent outcomes for patients and populations as a core part of clinicians' professional identity

code a set of symbols that are combined to build a communication message – for example, type of language or graphic representations

communication models ways of describing communication in a diagrammatic form – for example, the linear, interactive and transaction models

competence the ability to consistently function safely and effectively as a registered nurse

congruent leadership when a leader establishes a match (or congruence) between their values and beliefs and their actions

context the time, place and relationship of something, which can determine the meaning of communication

critical digital literacy digital literacies with a focus on critical thinking skills

cultural practices the non-verbal and verbal behaviours and rituals that are shared by cultural groups or sub-groups

culture what people do every day: how they behave, speak, relate and make things

digital literacies the skill set needed to effectively use digital technologies in order to access, understand and participate in the digital world

emotional intelligence the emotional and social characteristics, skills and enablers that determine how we perceive and express ourselves, understand and relate to others, and cope with daily living

empathy understanding another person's point of view

evidence the information you have gathered to support each main point

evidence-based healthcare emphasises the use of evidence from well-designed and conducted research in healthcare decision-making

evidence-informed practice (EIP) ensuring health practice is guided by the best research and information available

haptics non-verbal communication relating to touch

healthcare team a group of people with common health goals and objectives, who work together to meet them

heterophilous the degree to which pairs of individuals who interact are different with respect to certain attributes, such as beliefs, values, education and social status

homophilous the degree to which pairs of individuals who interact are similar with respect to certain attributes, such as beliefs, values, education and social status

implementation science all aspects of research relevant to the scientific study of methods to promote the uptake of research findings into routine settings in clinical, community and policy contexts

information literacy a set of skills for searching for, locating, evaluating and using information

interpersonal barriers barriers between people, such as gender, status and culture

intranet an organisation's private network, based on internet technology and accessed via the internet; usually protected from unauthorised access by firewalls

intrapersonal/psychological barriers barriers within a person, such as bias, anxiety and assumptions, that impede communication

jargon refers to the meanings of words and technical or specialised language shared by a specific cultural group or sub-group

kinesics non-verbal behaviour relating to body movement (facial expressions, gestures, gesticulations and movement); body language

leadership undertaken or carried out by people who try to unify people around values and then construct the social world for others around those values

lifelong learning the ongoing, voluntary and self-motivated pursuit of

knowledge for personal or professional reasons

literacies the characteristics, understandings, expectations and ways of behaving or acting in a certain context or culture – for example, academic literacy and numeracy refer to the skills of being able to read, write and do maths

main points the reasons for supporting a thesis statement or the viewpoint or stance you have taken in relation to your writing task

management the process of leading and directing all or part of an organisation, through the deployment and manipulation of resources

media literacy the ability to decode, evaluate, analyse and produce messages in a wide variety of media formats

multiliteracies the skill set needed to create meaning in ways that are increasingly multimodal, and in which text interfaces with oral, visual, audio, gestural, tactile and spatial patterns of meaning

noise a communication theory term – any barrier that affects the transmission of a message

oculesics non-verbal communication relating to eye behaviour

organisation a collection of individuals brought together in a particular environment to achieve a set of pre-determined objectives

organisational culture reflects the norms or traditions of the organisation and is exemplified by behaviours that illustrate values and beliefs

paralinguistics the tone of voice that can convey a non-verbal message

personal disposition the predominant or prevailing tendency of one's own inclinations and preferences

physical barriers any environmental or resource issues that affect the physical comfort or health of people, ultimately weakening the communication process.

power relationships relationships between individuals with differing levels of power in a specific context

professional communication a process by which information, perception and understanding are transmitted from person to person

professional identity how an individual perceives and employs the characteristics that define their professional self

quality initiatives actions taken within the health-care system that strive to provide safe, high-quality healthcare, improve the patient experience, tackle effectiveness and update practice in the light of evidence from research

research utilisation the movement of innovative research evidence into practice

self-awareness an individual's insight into their own behaviour; acknowledging personal strengths and weaknesses

self-concept the way we view ourselves; self-concept is not necessarily accurate

self-efficacy self-belief in a person's strengths and abilities to achieve their goals

semantic barriers misunderstanding created by the use of words such as jargon or specialised language

social media websites and applications that enable users to share content and participate in social networking

thesis statement your viewpoint in relation to the writing task

validation accepting what another person says as being valid to improve the flow of communication

workplace bullying repeated aggressive behaviour against work colleagues

Index